MW00652182

# Genetic Epidemiology

## Methods and Applications

# Genetic Epidemiology

## Methods and Applications

**Melissa A. Austin**
*University of Washington*

**Terri H. Beaty**
*Johns Hopkins University*

**W. David Dotson**
*Centers for Disease Control and Prevention*

**Kelly Edwards**
*University of Washington*

**Stephanie M. Fullerton**
*University of Washington*

**Marta Gwinn**
*McKing Consulting Corporation*

**Muin J. Khoury**
*Centers for Disease Control and Prevention*

**Barbara McKnight**
*University of Washington*

**Ruth Ottman**
*Columbia University*

**Bruce M. Psaty**
*University of Washington*

**Stephen M. Schwartz**
*Fred Hutchinson Cancer Research Center*

**Janet L. Stanford**
*Fred Hutchinson Cancer Research Center*

**Timothy A. Thornton**
*University of Washington*

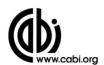

www.cabi.org

CABI is a trading name of CAB International

| | |
|---|---|
| CABI | CABI |
| Nosworthy Way | 38 Chauncey Street |
| Wallingford | Suite 1002 |
| Oxfordshire OX10 8DE | Boston, MA 02111 |
| UK | USA |
| | |
| Tel: +44 (0)1491 832111 | Tel: +1 800 552 3083 (toll free) |
| Fax: +44 (0)1491 833508 | Tel: +1 (0)617 395 4051 |
| E-mail: info@cabi.org | E-mail: cabi-nao@cabi.org |
| Website: www.cabi.org | |

© M.A. Austin 2013. All rights reserved. No part of this publication may be reproduced in any form or by any means, electronically, mechanically, by photocopying, recording or otherwise, without the prior permission of the copyright owners.

A catalogue record for this book is available from the British Library, London, UK.

**Library of Congress Cataloging-in-Publication Data**

Austin, Melissa A., author.
  Genetic epidemiology : methods and applications / Melissa A. Austin [and 12 others].
    p. ; cm. -- (Modular texts)
  Includes bibliographical references and index.
  ISBN 978-1-78064-181-2 (alk. paper)
  I. Title. II. Series: Modular texts.
  [DNLM: 1. Molecular Epidemiology. 2. Epidemiologic Methods. 3. Genetic Techniques. WA 950]

RB155
616'.042--dc23
                                        2013002766

ISBN: 978 1 78064 181 2

Commissioning editor: Rachel Cutts
Editorial assistant: Alexandra Lainsbury
Production editor: Tracy Head

Typeset by SPi, Pondicherry, India.
Printed and bound by Gutenberg Press Ltd, Tarxien, Malta.

# Contents

The color plates can be found following page 96.

# Contributors

**Melissa A. Austin, M.S., Ph.D.,** Department of Epidemiology, University of Washington, Seattle, Washington; E-mail: maustin@u.washington.edu

**Terri H. Beaty, Ph.D.,** Department of Epidemiology, Johns Hopkins University, Baltimore, Maryland; E-mail: tbeaty@jhsph.edu

**W. David Dotson, Ph.D.,** Office of Public Health Genomics, Centers for Disease Control and Prevention, Atlanta, Georgia; E-mail: gle1@cdc.gov

**Kelly Edwards, Ph.D.,** Department of Bioethics and Humanities, University of Washington, Seattle, Washington; E-mail: edwards@u.washington.edu

**Stephanie M. Fullerton, D.Phil.,** Department of Bioethics and Humanities, University of Washington, Seattle, Washington; E-mail: smfllrtn@u.washington.edu

**Marta Gwinn, M.D., M.P.H.,** McKing Consulting Corporation, Office of Public Health Genomics, Centers for Disease Control and Prevention, Atlanta, Georgia; E-mail: mlg1@cdc.gov

**Barbara McKnight, Ph.D.,** Department of Biostatistics, University of Washington, Seattle, Washington; E-mail: bmck@u.washington.edu

**Ruth Ottman, Ph.D.,** G.H. Sergievsky Center and Departments of Epidemiology and Neurology, Columbia University, New York; E-mail: ro6@cumc.columbia.edu

**Bruce M. Psaty, M.D., Ph.D.,** Cardiovascular Health Research Unit, Departments of Medicine, Epidemiology, and Health Services, University of Washington and Group Health Research Institute, Group Health Cooperative, Seattle, Washington; E-mail: psaty@u.washington.edu

**Stephen M. Schwartz, Ph.D., M.P.H.,** Division of Public Health Sciences, Fred Hutchinson Cancer Research Center, and Department of Epidemiology, University of Washington, Seattle, Washington; E-mail: stevesch@u.washington.edu

**Janet L. Stanford, M.P.H., Ph.D.,** Division of Public Health Sciences, Fred Hutchinson Cancer Research Center, and Department of Epidemiology, University of Washington, Seattle, Washington; E-mail: jstanford@fhcrc.org

**Timothy A. Thornton, Ph.D.,** Department of Biostatistics, University of Washington, Seattle, Washington; E-mail: tathornt@u.washington.edu

# Foreword

What a difference 20 years can make! Since the publication of *Fundamentals of Genetic Epidemiology* in 1993, genetic epidemiology has evolved from a relatively obscure scientific discipline to a mainstream field with real impact on medicine and public health. Prior to the genome era, the field consisted primarily of population and statistical geneticists, and a few epidemiologists interested in searching for the genetic basis of human disease. Today, the thriving field of genetic epidemiology is integrated into clinical and public health research. What has changed? The completion of the Human Genome Project and the initiatives and technologies that came along in the past decade have paved the way for increased sophistication in how we can approach the study of genetic factors and gene–environment interaction. Whole-genome sequencing and other "omic" fields are providing many tools for genetic epidemiology of the 21st century. Genetic Epidemiology with a capital E has truly arrived. In the face of all these changes, Melissa Austin has undertaken the formidable task of capturing the evolving field. Along with a few expert authors, she has applied a systematic approach to revisit the fundamentals of genetic epidemiology. The book tackles genetic concepts and technologies in relation to both population and family studies. It provides a sound methodological framework and covers the expanding array of tools, software, and data resources for the field. It goes over the ever more complicated landscape of gene–environment interaction. It addresses novel concepts of non-Mendelian genetics, such as epigenetics, that could prove crucial in our understanding of health and disease throughout the lifespan. The book describes thoroughly the ethical, legal, and social implications of the field. Finally, the book describes a translational framework for *how* to use emerging genetic epidemiologic information to improve health outcomes both at the individual and population levels. I am confident that the book will be a great resource for researchers, students, and practitioners from multiple scientific disciplines. Readers will gain valuable insight in approaches needed to identify the genomic foundation of human diseases and how to use this information to improve population health. We truly live in exciting times and I would not even want to guess where the field will be in another 20 years! Nevertheless, while the knowledge accrued from genomics and related fields will rapidly evolve, the fundamental genetic epidemiological principles for describing, evaluating, implementing, and monitoring this new knowledge will be with us for years to come.

**Muin J. Khoury**
Atlanta, Georgia
1 January 2013

# Acknowledgments

The authors would like to thank the following colleagues who contributed to this book by sharing material from their lectures and/or providing reviews: Roger Bumgarner, David L. Eaton, Susan R. Heckbert, Deborah A. Nickerson, and Bruce S. Weir from the University of Washington, Carolyn M. Hutter from the National Cancer Institute, and Sharon L.R. Kardia from the University of Michigan.

# 1 The Evolving Field of Genetic Epidemiology

Melissa A. Austin, M.S., Ph.D.[1]
and Terri H. Beaty, Ph.D.[2]

[1]Department of Epidemiology, University of Washington, Seattle, Washington; [2]Department of Epidemiology, Johns Hopkins University, Baltimore, Maryland

## 1.1 Introduction

Genetic epidemiology is an interdisciplinary field that has integrated human genetics and epidemiology for over 50 years (Beaty and Khoury, 2000). In their 1993 textbook, Khoury, Beaty, and Cohen listed no fewer than eight different definitions of genetic epidemiology, many of which describe studying the etiology of diseases in families and the inherited causes of disease in populations. For example, Rao (1984) emphasizes how genetic epidemiology differs from its parent disciplines: "... an emerging field ... that represents an important interaction between the two parent disciplines: genetics and epidemiology. Genetic epidemiology differs from epidemiology by its explicit consideration of genetic factors and family resemblance; it differs from population genetics by its focus on disease; it also differs from medical genetics by its emphasis on population aspects."

As shown in Table 1.1, the origins, focus, analytic tools, and goals of genetics and epidemiology differ. However, public health researchers, medical geneticists, and genome scientists all realize the importance of integrating these two disciplines to advance our understanding of health and disease in both families and populations.

In the same textbook, Khoury *et al.* (1993) thoroughly described the fundamental principles of genetic epidemiology research. The field has expanded and broadened during the past 20 years, although these principles remain relevant to ongoing studies of genetic susceptibility to disease in populations. Public health researchers now recognize the importance of genetic factors in disease susceptibility. The remarkable advances in genetics and genetic epidemiology have led to the discovery of thousands of genetic variants showing consistent association with both common, complex disease and hundreds of variants/mutations controlling rare, Mendelian disorders. As recently stated by the National Human Genome Research Institute (NHGRI) (Green *et al.*, 2011), "Opportunities for understanding health and disease are now unprecedented, as advances in genomics are harnessed to obtain robust foundational knowledge about the structure and function of the human genome and about the genetic contributions to human health and disease." This progress is due to many factors, including innovations in genomic technology, statistical and computational developments, and the availability of DNA samples and epidemiologic data for harmonized phenotypes from large population-based studies. Internet-based communication and data sharing have enhanced collaboration between investigators for large-scale studies, providing the large sample sizes

© M.A. Austin 2013. *Genetic Epidemiology: Methods and Applications*
(M.A. Austin *et al.*)

**Table 1.1.** Comparison of genetics and epidemiology.

|  | Genetics | Epidemiology |
|---|---|---|
| Origins | Biological science of inheritance<br>Experimental/breeding | Methodological science of public health<br>Observational/analytic studies |
| Focus | Mechanisms of inheritance, often<br>on rare diseases | Etiologic factors, primarily on common<br>diseases |
| Tools | Family studies<br>Laboratory methods<br>Statistical models<br>Population models | Observational studies<br>Case–control studies<br>Cohort designs<br>Clinical trials |
| Goals | Understand mechanisms of<br>inheritance | Understand distribution, etiology, and<br>progression of disease |
| Overlap | Diseases of interest<br>Population studies<br>Ultimate goal of disease prevention ||

needed to detect modest effects of individual genes for diseases controlled by multiple genes and environmental risk factors together. Web-based software and data resources have also become essential tools in genetic epidemiology research.

In this textbook, we strive to explain and illustrate the fundamental principles of genetic epidemiology research in the context of the rapid changes in the field. Each description of a study design or approach is illustrated with relevant applications from the literature. In the following overview, we provide a summary of each of the topics covered in this book, their current relevance to genetic epidemiology, and how they continue to evolve.

## 1.2   Assessing Genetic Influences on Disease, Human Genetics Concepts, and Genomic Technology

In Chapters 2 and 3 of this textbook, we lay the foundation for genetic epidemiology research methods. We begin by emphasizing the necessity of determining the magnitude of genetic influences on the disease, risk factor, or trait of interest using familial aggregation and/or heritability analysis. This is important for two reasons. First, if there is little or no genetic influence on a disease of interest, genetic epidemiology studies to identify the genes involved are unlikely to be successful or at least will be more difficult. Although this may seem obvious, it is easy to overlook this step in the excitement of applying new genomic technologies to address innovative research hypotheses. Secondly, once disease susceptibility genes have been identified, these initial analyses can be used to determine the degree to which the identified genetic variants can explain the underlying genetic predisposition.

More specifically, the goal of familial aggregation analysis is to determine if a disease occurs more frequently among relatives of an affected individual than in the general population, which can reflect the presence of genetic influences on disease. Heritability has a very specific meaning in genetic epidemiology, and is often misunderstood. Heritability is defined as the proportion of the variance in a quantitative phenotype or in risk for disease that is attributable to unspecified genes under a polygenic model, where many independent genes (each with small, additive effects) determine the phenotype along with an independent environmental component. As such, heritability estimates (which range from 0 to 1) do not provide information about biological mechanisms, but do offer a simple quantitative measure of the degree of genetic control. Heritability is often estimated by comparing monozygous and dizygous twins, but other relatives can be used. It is important to keep in mind that many assumptions must be made in this type of analysis, some of which are easily tested and some of which are not. The concepts of polygenic inheritance and heritability were developed nearly a century ago, long before the availability of genomic data. They have, however, taken on new importance in the context of genome-wide association studies and DNA sequencing studies, as will be described in Chapter 5.

Next, we provide a brief review of basic concepts in human genetics. This is not intended to be comprehensive, and readers are encouraged to refer to established texts referenced in Chapter 3, especially for new genetic concepts. This chapter is organized to focus first on concepts related to single genes, then to principles related to multiple genes. Concepts related to single genes include: Mendelian inheritance, modes of inheritance, the Online Mendelian Inheritance in Man (OMIM®) resource, a description of the characteristics of complex genetic traits, the Hardy–Weinberg principle, the genetic code, basic gene structure, types of genetic markers including single nucleotide polymorphisms (SNPs) and copy number variants (CNVs), and the concept of identify by descent (IBD). Concepts related to multiple genes include: genetic linkage, recombination, linkage disequilibrium (LD), haplotypes, and tag SNPs.

Chapter 3 includes a summary of recent advances in genomic technology, with an emphasis on their relevance to genetic epidemiology. This overview describes genome-wide SNP genotyping platforms and presents the basic steps in three generations of DNA sequencing (Sanger sequencing, "next-generation" or massively parallel DNA sequencing methods, and "single molecule systems" that are under development) and in exome sequencing. The importance of quality control and potential sources of bias in sequencing data are also described. Chapter 3 concludes with a summary of study designs for common and rare genetic variants.

## 1.3  Family-based Study Designs: Linkage, Exome Sequencing, and Case–Parent Trios

Since the inception of the field, family studies have been a fundamental research method in genetic epidemiology for mapping disease susceptibility genes (Wang *et al.*, 2010). In Chapter 4, we describe the basics of LOD score linkage analysis, a traditional research method comparing the number of recombinant and non-recombinant offspring in families to search for evidence of co-segregation between a hypothetical disease gene and a known genetic marker. Interpretation of findings from linkage analysis is straightforward because there is a solid biological basis behind these statistics: recombination during meiosis. This approach generally works best for rare, Mendelian disorders, using multigenerational families containing many affected members. Non-parametric linkage analysis, which uses excess sharing of marker alleles IBD, especially between siblings, is an alternative approach for linkage analysis which builds upon smaller families that are easier to find and recruit.

During the last two decades, family studies in genetic epidemiology have evolved from using linkage analysis to exome sequencing for mapping disease susceptibility genes. Such studies are providing major advances in our understanding of genetic susceptibility to rare, familial forms of disease, as well as common, complex diseases. We illustrate with examples from research on familial breast cancer, familial pancreatic cancer, and familial prostate cancer.

Unlike linkage studies, genetic association studies typically test for differences in allele, genotype, or haplotype frequencies between groups of unrelated individuals (such as cases and controls). However, genetic association studies can also be conducted in families using parent–offspring trios. These family-based tests of association compare the observed frequency of transmission of a marker allele from parents to an affected offspring with the expected frequency based on strict Mendelian inheritance. The transmission disequilibrium test (TDT) is one of the original such tests, and actually tests a composite null hypothesis of no linkage or no linkage disequilibrium.

## 1.4 Genetic Association Studies of Common and Rare Variants, Large-scale Collaborations, and Population Stratification

Based on the "common disease/common variant" hypothesis proposed in the early 1990s, genetic epidemiologists have undertaken genetic association studies of unrelated individuals to search for susceptibility genes for many complex diseases, using either candidate gene or genome-wide approaches. In the candidate gene approach, genes whose functions are known (or suspected) to be involved in disease predisposition, and specific polymorphisms within those genes, are studied. Genome-wide association studies (GWAS) do not rely on known etiologic mechanisms and examine genetic markers spanning the entire genome to identify new genes or confirm previously known susceptibility genes. They use high-throughput technologies for genotyping millions of SNPs on each sample. To have sufficient statistical power to detect the small effect sizes found in most GWAS, very large samples are needed, and are often based on large-scale collaborations involving multiple studies. Chapter 5 describes methods for both approaches using case–control, cohort, and case–parent trio study designs.

Unlike genetic linkage studies, interpretation of genetic association results is complex and such associations can be attributable to a direct, causal relationship between an observed marker and an unobserved causal gene, or an indirect relationship reflecting linkage disequilibrium between the observed marker and the unobserved causal gene. False-positive associations are a concern in genetic association studies because of the large number of statistical tests, each with some probability of error, so issues of multiple comparisons, departures of genetic markers from the Hardy–Weinberg equilibrium, and/or population stratification must always be considered carefully. Chapter 6 emphasizes that analysis of GWAS data should always include evaluation of the possible role of confounding owing to population stratification, and when it is present, use available statistical methods to control it. This needs to include an evaluation of both "global" population stratification occurring when subgroups of the study population have a distinct ancestry associated with both marker allele frequencies and baseline differences in disease risk, and "local" structure detectable

M.A. Austin and T.H. Beaty

in recently admixed populations. Finally, false negatives are also possible in genetic association studies and these can reflect inadequate statistical power, small effect sizes, and/or insufficient genomic coverage in the particular marker panel used.

The Cohorts for Heart and Aging Research in Genomic Epidemiology (CHARGE) Consortium is an example of an effective and productive GWAS collaboration that takes advantage of large sample sizes from existing cohort studies, and provides a model for investigator-initiated collaborative research to identify genetic markers associated with a variety of cardiovascular and aging phenotypes.

Although more than 2,000 SNPs have been associated with complex traits and diseases to date based on GWAS, these documented associations cannot explain most of the heritability of these traits, i.e. even when multiple markers are confirmed to be associated with a complex phenotype, simply summing their estimated effects generally does not approach the overall summary estimate of heritability. Using height as an example, possible reasons for this "missing heritability" are considered, and demonstrate the need for very large sample sizes in GWAS.

More recently, the alternative "common disease/rare variant" (CDRV) hypothesis has been proposed. Rather than complex diseases being completely explained through association with multiple markers, each with a small effect on risk, this theory proposes that common diseases are due to effects of multiple rare, deleterious variants each with a strong impact on risk. DNA sequence data, including exome sequencing results, are capable of addressing the CDRV hypothesis. Implementing new genetic epidemiology study designs, including sequencing affected relatives in families with multiple affected individuals or individuals drawn from the extremes of a phenotype distribution, holds the potential to identify causal genes under this hypothesis. Statistical methods for discovering associations of rare genetic variants with disease risk are fundamentally different from statistics used to discover associations with common genetic variants, and these methods are also developing rapidly. These "burden tests" combine all the different rare variants in a gene, a biological pathway, or a regulatory region, and incorporate functional genetic data into their analysis to identify causal variants.

## 1.5   Gene–Environment Interactions, Epistasis, and Non-Mendelian Genetics

Understanding the role of gene–environment and gene–gene interactions (epistasis) in disease susceptibility can increase the statistical power, accuracy, and precision for detecting genetic and environmental effects, as well as improving our understanding of biological mechanisms of disease risk.

In Chapter 7, we begin by presenting five biologically plausible models of relationships between a genotype and an exposure and their combined effect on disease risk, to conceptualize different types of interaction. Next, we explain the use of an additive or multiplicative measurement scale in evaluating such interactions, and describe causal modeling approaches from epidemiology that can be used to address this problem.

The case-only study design is a useful approach for evaluating interactions, and can provide greater statistical power than the standard case–control method under certain circumstances. In this approach, association between the potential susceptibility genotype and the exposure of interest are tested only among cases. This method, however, relies on the assumption that genetic and environmental risk factors occur independently, and it can only test for interaction on a multiplicative scale.

One of the most important, emerging areas for the study of gene–environment interaction is pharmacogenomics, the study of genotypes controlling efficacy and adverse effects of medications. Findings from many such ongoing studies have important implications for "personalized medicine" and public health, and to date have focused primarily on approved prescription drugs. In this chapter, Chapter 7, we present the example of carbamazepine, a medication approved for the treatment of epilepsy, bipolar I disorders, trigeminal neuralgia, and more general neuropathic pain, and its association with serious and sometimes fatal dermatological reactions such as Stevens–Johnson syndrome (SJS) and toxic epidermal necrolysis (TEN).

The remarkable success of GWAS has created unprecedented opportunities for studying the role of gene–environment interactions in disease risk by integrating associations found in GWAS with environmental risk factors. These emerging types of studies have been termed gene–environment-wide interaction studies or GEWIS. They provide opportunities both for identifying gene–environment interactions by building on existing GWAS results, and for discovering new susceptibility variants that are not identified in studies that only consider marginal genetic effects. One of the major challenges for such studies is the harmonization of previously collected environmental data, usually from many collaborating studies, because environmental phenotypes may have been obtained using different questionnaires and data collection methods. The growing interest in GEWIS studies has also spurred the development of new statistical methods to characterize gene–environment interactions in the context of genome-wide data, including hybrid methods combining case–control and case-only analysis results.

Lastly in Chapter 7, we discuss the importance of taking into account epistasis for understanding genetic pathways and improving detection of genetic influences on complex diseases. Similar to the concepts of multiplicative and additive scales of interaction described above, there are also several definitions of epistasis based on differing statistical and biological models, and new statistical methods are under development, particularly for use with GWAS data.

In Chapter 8, we turn to non-Mendelian genetics, including mitochondrial DNA variation, parental and parent-of-origin effects, *de novo* variation, and epigenetic factors (heritable characteristics of chromosomes other than DNA sequence variation that influence gene expression). These mechanisms have been primarily examined in either rare conditions or a small subset of common conditions, and determining whether non-Mendelian effects account for a measurable proportion of common, complex diseases will require both innovative study designs and statistical methods, and must consider the most appropriate sources of DNA.

## 1.6  Software and Data Resources

One of the most important advances in genetic epidemiology during the last 15 years has been the development of a remarkable array of web-based resources that have become available for genetic epidemiologists. These include extensive statistical software, genomic databases containing genotype and phenotype data, and population reference panels with high-throughput SNP genotyping and next-generation sequencing data either freely available or through monitored access. In Chapter 9, we provide information about navigating these resources, including guidance for finding appropriate software for the analysis of data and identifying and gaining access to suitable genetic data.

Software resources available for genetic epidemiology studies include: R, a free software environment for statistics and graphics; PLINK, a free, open-source software designed to perform a range of analyses for large-scale genetic data; software to account for population structure in genetic association studies, to estimate ancestry, and for genetic relatedness inference; software for power calculations and for imputation of untyped genetic markers; and a comprehensive alphabetical list of genetic analysis software. Human reference panels and resources include: HapMap; the Human Genetics Diversity Panel (HGDP); 1000 Genomes Project; and the Genome Variation Server. Genotype and phenotype repositories include the database of Genotypes and Phenotypes (dbGaP) and the European Genome-Phenome Archive (EGA). We highlight the usefulness of these resources and provide two examples to illustrate how these data and software resources can be used, one characterizing patterns of linkage disequilibrium and another estimating ancestry.

## 1.7   Ethical Issues and Translational Genetic Epidemiology

Genetic epidemiology studies require the voluntary participation of both patients and healthy individuals, whose genomic and phenotypic data are essential for advancing scientific discovery. In Chapter 10, we describe how this creates researcher–participant interactions that create a host of important regulatory and ethical concerns that should be addressed at the earliest stages of designing and implementing a program of research.

All such research involving living human subjects is guided by a set of federal regulations known as "the Common Rule," which are based on three core ethical principles: Respect for Persons, Beneficence, and Justice. Respect for Persons is operationalized as informed consent to participate in research. Ideally, participants should understand the nature of the study, the likely risks, benefits, and uncertainties, and that their participation is voluntary. Beneficence is maximizing good outcomes for humanity and research subjects, while minimizing or avoiding risks or harm. Justice is ensuring reasonable, non-exploitative, and well-considered procedures are administered fairly (the fair distribution of costs and benefits).

Recent research has demonstrated that participants may value having a say in research decision making, especially where future uses of data and specimens are difficult to predict at the time of their initial recruitment. In biomedical research, governance typically means giving attention to these decision-making processes and structures throughout the course of specimen or data collection, handling, distribution, and use. Elements of research governance for a genetic epidemiology study include participant recruitment, data storage and management, consent, data access, return of results to participants, communication, and oversight. New adaptive approaches to research governance may provide a more effective way of maximizing secondary uses of specimens and data while respecting participants' altruistic contributions to research.

We conclude the textbook with a discussion of public health and clinical applications of genetic epidemiology, i.e. translating findings from genetic epidemiology research studies to clinical practice and improved public health outcomes. In particular, public health has an interest in ensuring the proposed applications of genomic research are scientifically valid and that they add value to existing practice and programs. In Chapter 11, we describe a four-phase translational framework: T1: Discovery to candidate health application; T2: Health application to evidence-based guidelines; T3: Guidelines to health practice; and T4: Practice to population health impact. Each of these phases is illustrated using cascade screening for Lynch syndrome to demonstrate that genetic epidemiology research presents new opportunities to bridge clinical medicine with public health.

## 1.8 Conclusion

In this chapter, we have provided an overview of the evolving field of genetic epidemiology, and briefly described the structure of this textbook. We have emphasized the ongoing developments in research methodology and the use of emerging technologies to better understand health and disease in families and populations. It is our hope this book with be useful for graduate students in public health who are motivated to improve population health by successfully integrating genetics and epidemiology into their own work.

## Further Reading

The 1000 Genomes Consortium (2010) A map of human genome variation from population-scale sequencing. *Nature* 467, 1061–1073.

Bamshad, M.J., Ng, S.B., Bigham, A.W., Tabor, H.K., Emond, M.J., Nickerson, D.A. and Shendure J. (2011) Exome sequencing as a tool for Mendelian Disease gene discovery. *Nature Reviews Genetics* 12, 745–755.

Belmont Report (1979) The Belmont Report: ethical principles and guidelines for the protection of human subjects of research. Available from: http://www.hhs.gov/ohrp/humansubjects/guidance/belmont.html (accessed August 21, 2012).

The ENCODE Project Consortium (2012) An integrated encyclopedia of DNA elements in the human genome. *Nature* 489, 57–74.

The International HapMap 3 Consortium (2010) Integrating common and rare genetic variation in diverse human populations. *Nature* 467, 52–58.

Khoury, M.J., Bedrosian, S.R., Gwinn, M., Higgins, J.P.T., Ioannidis, J.P.A. and Little, J. (eds) (2010) *Human Genome Epidemiology: Building the Evidence for Using Genetic Information to Improve Health and Prevent Disease*, 2nd edn. Oxford University Press, New York. Selected chapters available at: http://www.cdc.gov/genomics/resources/books/2010_HuGE/index.htm (accessed July 19, 2012).

Manolio, T.A. (2010) Genomewide association studies and assessment of the risk of disease. *New England Journal of Medicine* 363, 166–176.

Novembre, J., Johnson, T., Bryc, K., Kutalik, Z., Boyko, A.R., Auton, A., *et al.* (2008) Genes mirror geography within Europe. *Nature* 456, 98–101.

Ott, J. (1999) *Analysis of Human Genetic Linkage*, 3rd edn. The Johns Hopkins University Press, Baltimore and London.

M.A. Austin and T.H. Beaty

Speicher, M.R., Antonarakis, S.E. and Motulsky A.G. (2010) *Vogel and Motulsky's Human Genetics. Problems and Approaches*, 4th edn. Springer-Verlag, Berlin, Germany.

Thomas, D. (2010) Gene-environment-wide association studies: emerging concepts. *Nature Reviews Genetics* 11, 259–272.

Visscher, P.M., Hill, W.G. and Wray, N.R. (2008) Heritability in the genomics era – concepts and misconceptions. *Nature Reviews Genetics* 9, 255–266.

# References

Beaty, T.H. and Khoury, M.J. (2000) Interface of genetics and epidemiology. *Epidemiologic Reviews* 22, 120–125.

Green, E.D., Guyer M.S. and National Human Genome Research Institute (2011) Charting a course for genomic medicine from base pairs to bedside. *Nature* 470, 204–213.

Khoury, M.J., Beaty, T.H. and Cohen, B.H. (1993) Epidemiologic approaches to familial aggregation. In: *Fundamentals of Genetic Epidemiology*. Oxford University Press, New York, pp. 164–199.

Rao, D.C. (1984) Editorial comment. *Genetic Epidemiology* 1, 5–6.

Wang, S.S., Beaty, T.H. and Khoury, M.J. (2010) Genetic epidemiology. In: Speicher, M.R., Antonarakis, S.E. and Motulsky, A.G. (eds) *Vogel and Motulsky's Human Genetics. Problems and Approaches*, 4th edn. Springer-Verlag, Berlin, Germany, pp. 617–634.

# 2  Assessing Genetic Influences on Diseases and Risk Factors

MELISSA A. AUSTIN, M.S., PH.D.

*Department of Epidemiology, University of Washington, Seattle, Washington*

## Synopsis

- Before applying advances in genomic technology to mapping genes for disease susceptibility, it is crucial to establish that genetic factors influence the disease or risk factor of interest.
- Familial aggregation analysis, used to determine if a disease occurs more frequently among relatives than in the general population, can reflect the presence of genetic influences on disease.
- Heritability has a very specific meaning in genetic epidemiology and is defined as the proportion of the variance in a disease or risk factor that is attributable to genetic influences under a polygenic model of many genes, each with small, additive effect on risk.
- Heritability is often estimated by comparing monozygous and dizygous twins, although many assumptions must be made in this analysis, and it should be interpreted carefully.
- The concepts of polygenic inheritance and heritability were developed nearly a century ago, but have taken on new importance in the context of genome-wide association studies.

## 2.1  Introduction

Although the primary emphasis of genetic epidemiology is to identify genes for human diseases and risk factors, an important first step is to insure that the trait of interest is genetically influenced. If there is little, if any, genetic contribution to a trait, it may not be possible to identify genes that contribute to it. If the trait is, in fact, genetically influenced, it is also important to estimate the magnitude of the genetic contribution. In this way, when genes are found to be linked or associated with the trait, it is possible to determine how much of the genetic contribution can be explained by these variants.

This chapter will focus on two approaches to characterize whether or not there are genetic influences on a disease or risk factor of interest: familial aggregation studies and estimating heritability using twin studies.

## 2.2  Familial Aggregation Studies

As the name implies, familial aggregation can be defined as "The occurrence of a disorder at a higher frequency in relatives of affected persons than in the general

© M.A. Austin 2013. *Genetic Epidemiology: Methods and Applications*
(M.A. Austin *et al.*)

population, whether for genetic or environmental reasons or both" (Susser and Susser, 1989). If familial aggregation of a disease is found, there are several possible explanations that must be kept in mind:

- *Genetic inheritance of the disease*
  This could be due to a single major gene effect or polygenic inheritance, or both.
- *Familial aggregation of risk factors related to the disease, rather than the disease itself*
  For example, there may be common environmental exposures among relatives living in the same household that increase their risk of disease, there could be cultural inheritance (traits that are passed from one generation to the next due only to cultural influences), and/or genetic inheritance of risk factors for the disease.
- *Gene–environment interactions*
  Genetic susceptibility among family members may interact with environmental influences that they also share to increase risk of disease.
- *Bias or confounding*
  Difference in family size between cases and controls, ascertainment bias, recall bias, and/or underlying disease heterogeneity can create a spurious appearance of familial aggregation of disease.
- *Statistical false positive*
  As with any statistical test, a type I error can lead to an incorrect inference, in this case that the disease clusters in families.

These points illustrate that familial aggregation can be consistent with the presence of genetic influences on a disease or risk factor, and thus provide preliminary evidence supporting a search for the genes involved. However, the possibility that other factors may be operating must always be considered as well.

### 2.2.1 Familial aggregation study designs

As shown in Table 2.1, there are two basic study designs to assess familial aggregation of a disease or risk factor from an epidemiologic perspective. This is because data collection for a family study usually begins with a group of "probands" with the disorder of interest. Such a group can be considered "cases" in the context of a family case–control study or, alternatively, can be considered an "exposure" for his or her relatives in what has been termed the "family cohort" approach. In this context, the "cohort" consists of relatives of the cases and controls. Both study designs require collecting data on disease occurrence among cases and controls, and their relatives. However, the hypotheses being tested differ, as do the statistical analyses.

In the family case–control approach, the hypothesis is: Is a family history of disease associated with increased risk of disease? The "population at risk" in this analysis is the cases and controls, the "exposure" is family history of disease, and the sample size (n) is the number of cases and controls. The data is tabulated as shown in Table 2.1A, and an odds ratio (OR = ad/bc) is calculated to estimate the magnitude of the association (Khoury *et al.*, 1993). As illustrated in Box 2.1, standard epidemiologic analyses can be applied, including adjusting for potential confounding factors (Breslow and Day, 1980).

**Table 2.1.** Study designs for familial aggregation studies (adapted from Khoury et al., 1993).

**A** "Family case–control" approach

| | Family history of disease | | |
| --- | --- | --- | --- |
| | Yes | No | Total |
| Number of cases | a | b | a + b |
| Number of controls | c | d | c + d |
| Total | | | n = number of cases and controls |

**B** "Family cohort" approach

| | Relative has disease | | |
| --- | --- | --- | --- |
| | Yes | No | Total |
| Number of relatives of cases | A | B | A + B |
| Number of relatives of controls | C | C | C + D |
| Total | | | N = number of relatives |

The investigator should carefully consider the definition of "family history" in this context to insure that it is appropriate for the disease under study. For example, in a study of ovarian cancer, family history should only include female relatives of the cases and controls. For late-onset diseases, offspring may be too young to have experienced the disease and may not be appropriate to include in the definition of family history.

In the "family cohort approach," the hypothesis is: Are relatives of cases with disease at increased risk compared with relatives of controls? In this setting, the "population at risk" is the relatives of the cases and controls, whereas the cases and controls represent exposure or lack of exposure, respectively. Thus, the sample size (N) consists of the number of relatives, and the relative risk (RR) = (A/(A+B))/(C/(C+D)) (Table 2.1B).

For either approach, a sample of cases with disease and a sample of controls are collected, and information on their family history of disease is ascertained. Ideally, such a study design would involve contacting appropriate relatives of the cases and controls individually and determining whether or not they also have the disease. Obtaining medical records would further insure that the diagnosis of relatives is accurate. However, because this is often not feasible owing to limited resources, researchers usually obtain family history data by interviewing the cases and controls. If this is done carefully, it can provide the necessary data for a familial aggregation analysis. To insure accurate data collection, family history interviews are often conducted in two stages. First, the study participant is asked to identify all the relevant relatives in his or her family. If the investigator is interested in first-degree relatives, the study participant would be asked to identify his or her parents, brothers and sisters, and any children, insuring that these relatives are biologically related. In the second stage of the interview, the investigator reviews the list of relatives with the study participant, asking if each one has the disease of interest.

## Box 2.1. Application: Family History of Pancreatic Cancer

Pancreatic cancer is the fourth leading cause of cancer mortality among both men and women in the USA. Most tumors are ductal adenocarcinoma of the pancreas and have a median survival of only 4 months (Fesinmeyer *et al.*, 2005). The inaccessibility of the pancreas, the non-specific symptoms of pancreatic cancer, and the resulting diagnosis at advanced stages of disease make etiologic studies of pancreatic cancer challenging.

It has been estimated that 5–10% of pancreatic cancer is genetically influenced (Brand and Lynch, 2006). Several studies have proposed candidate genes for risk of pancreatic cancer, including an exomic sequencing study showing that mutations in the *PALB2* gene are responsible for a hereditary form of the disease (Jones *et al.*, 2009) (see Box 4.1), and recent studies that have identified an association between the ABO locus on chromosome 9 and risk of pancreatic cancer (Amundadottir *et al.*, 2009; Wolpin *et al.*, 2009) (see Box 5.3).

A meta-analysis of nine epidemiologic studies reported a weighted, adjusted overall RR of 1.80 (95% CI 1.48–2.12) of pancreatic cancer associated with having an affected relative (Permuth-Wey and Egan, 2009), but the magnitude of the association is not well established. To address this question, Jacobs *et al.* (2010) used data from the Pancreatic Cancer Cohort Consortium (PanScan) to assess the association between having a family history of pancreatic cancer in a first-degree relative and the risk of pancreatic cancer.

### Study design and data analysis

PanScan, which was created to conduct a genome-wide association study, included cases and matched controls from 12 prospective cohort studies and one "ultra rapid" case–control study from the USA, Europe and China. The family history of pancreatic cancer analysis included seven of these studies with a total of 1,183 cases and 1,205 controls.

Eligible cases for the study were incident pancreatic ductal adenocarcinoma cases confirmed through cancer registries, death certificates, or review of medical records. Controls were matched to cases based on year of birth, sex, and race, and other factors in some studies, and were alive at the incidence date for the matched case.

Family history data were collected using self-reported, written questionnaires. The analysis presented by Jacobs *et al.* (2010) only considered family history in first-degree relatives, including parents, siblings, and offspring. In addition to dichotomizing on family history as "yes/no," the authors examined the number of affected relatives and the age at diagnosis of the youngest affected relative. ORs and 95% CIs were calculated using unconditional logistic regression, adjusted for age, study, sex, smoking, race, and self-reported diabetes.

### Family case–control study results for pancreatic cancer

As shown in Table 2.2, the association between a family history of pancreatic cancer in a first-degree relative and risk of pancreatic cancer was moderate (OR = 1.76), although

*Continued*

Box 2.1. *Continued.*

**Table 2.2.** Association between family history of pancreatic cancer and risk of pancreatic cancer (adapted from Jacobs *et al.*, 2010).

| | No. of cases (%) | No. of controls (%) | Adjusted OR[a] | 95% CI |
|---|---|---|---|---|
| Family history of pancreatic cancer in 1st-degree relative | | | | |
| No | 1,107 (93.6) | 1,162 (96.4) | 1.0 (ref) | (1.19–2.61) |
| Yes | 76 (6.4) | 43 (3.6) | 1.76 | |
| Number of affected 1st-degree relatives with pancreatic cancer | | | | |
| One | 70 (92.1) | 42 (97.7) | 1.70 | (1.14–2.53) |
| Two or more | 6 (7.9) | 1 (2.3) | 4.26 | (0.48–37.79) |
| Age at diagnosis of youngest affected 1st-degree relative | | | | |
| ≥60 years | 38 (65.5) | 22 (66.7) | 1.82 | (1.05–3.13) |
| <60 years | 20 (34.5) | 11 (33.3) | 1.54 | (0.71–3.34) |

[a]Adjusted for sex, study, smoking, race, and diabetes.

statistically significant. ORs in the individual studies ranged from 0.38 to 3.54. Because having two or more affected relatives was rare, this association could not be accurately assessed, resulting in a very wide CI (0.48–37.79). Similar ORs were seen for age of diagnosis of the youngest affected relative ≥60 or <60 years (1.82 and 1.54, respectively). Taken together, the results indicate an approximately twofold increased risk for pancreatic cancer associated with a first-degree relative family history of pancreatic cancer, similar to previous studies. The data also provide evidence to justify studies to understand the extent to which this association is due to genetic influences.

It is important to keep in mind that there are, however, many potential sources of bias in such an interview process. For example, if cases are from larger families than controls, the probability of a case having a relative affected with the disease is higher than controls. There may also be differential recall between cases and controls, especially for more distant relatives. That is, a family with several cases of disease, or a pair of affected twins, may tend to attract more interest, and thus better recall than a family with less disease experience. However, once the family history data are collected, both approaches can be applied to the same data set, allowing a comparison of the results using two different analyses.

## 2.3 Heritability Analysis

Although the term "heritability" is widely used in genetic epidemiology, it has a specific statistical meaning that is based on an additive polygenic model, and on partitioning the variance of a disease or risk factor into genetic and environmental components

(Visscher *et al.*, 2008). That is, the value of a phenotype P (either continuous or dichotomous) can be expressed as:

$$P = \mu + G + E$$

where $\mu$ is the mean, G are genetic effects, and E are environmental effects. It then follows that the variance of P can be written as:

$$\sigma^2_P = \sigma^2_G + \sigma^2_E$$

And the "broad sense" heritability of P is defined as:

$$H^2 = \sigma^2_G / \sigma^2_P$$

That is, the heritability $H^2$ is the proportion of the variance in P that is attributable to genetic influences. $H^2$ ranges from 0 (little or no genetic influence) to 1 (strong genetic influences).

The genetic component of the variance can be further partitioned into additive effects (A), representing the effects of many genes, each with a small, additive effect, and dominance effects (D) between alleles at each locus. So:

$$\sigma^2_G = \sigma^2_A + \sigma^2_D$$

and the "narrow sense" heritability is defined by:

$$h^2 = \sigma^2_A / \sigma^2_P$$

while the "broad sense" heritability can be expressed as:

$$H^2 = (\sigma^2_A + \sigma^2_D) / \sigma^2_P$$

### 2.3.1 Polygenic model

In addition to depending on a simple linear model, the genetic component of heritability analysis is based on a polygenic model using the "liability scale" (Falconer, 1965). To illustrate this model, assume that there are two unlinked genes contributing to the phenotype P, each with two alleles: gene 1 with allele A and a, and gene 2 with alleles B and b. Under this model, each capital letter allele increases an individual's risk of disease by 1 unit on the liability scale. If the trait is dichotomous, a threshold value Z is assumed, such that individuals with a liability score above this value express the disease.

Under this model, each possible genotype, the corresponding liability score, and the frequency of each genotype are listed in Table 2.3.

**Table 2.3.** Genotypes, liability scores, and genotype frequencies under a polygenic model with two loci.

| Genotype(s) | Liability score | Frequency |
| --- | --- | --- |
| aabb | 0 | 1 |
| Aabb, aAbb, aaBb, aabB | +1 | 4 |
| AAbb, AaBb, AabB, aABb, aAbB, aaBB | +2 | 6 |
| AABb, AAbB, AaBB, aABB | +3 | 4 |
| AABB | +4 | 1 |

By plotting the frequency of genotypes by liability score, the resulting distribution (Fig. 2.1) approximates a normal, Gaussian distribution.

If we then assume that there are three loci contributing to the heritability of the trait of interest, with the addition of alleles C and c for the third gene, we can again tabulate the possible genotypes and corresponding liability scores (Table 2.4).

As shown in Fig. 2.2, we again see an approximate Gaussian distribution for the frequency of genotypes by liability score. If our trait is dichotomous, a threshold value Z determines the liability score above which an individual is affected.

We could continue this exercise with any number of genes contributing to the trait under the polygenic model and would always find a similar distribution. Thus, the value of this model is that one can estimate heritability without knowledge of the number of genes involved, as long as an additive model is assumed.

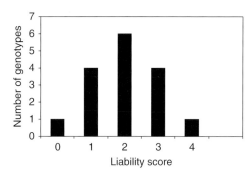

**Fig. 2.1.** Frequency distribution of genotypes by liability score under a polygenic model with two loci.

**Table 2.4.** Genotypes, liability scores, and genotype frequencies under a polygenic model with three loci.

| Genotype(s) | Liability score | Frequency |
| --- | --- | --- |
| aabbcc | 0 | 1 |
| Aabbcc, aAbbcc, aaBbcc, aabBcc, aabbCc, aabbcC | +1 | 6 |
| AAbbcc, AaBbcc, AabBcc, … | +2 | 15 |
| AABbcc, AAbBcc, AaBBcc, … | +3 | 20 |
| AABBcc, AABbCc, AABbcC, … | +4 | 15 |
| AABBCc, AABBcC, AABbCC, … | +5 | 6 |
| AABBCC | +6 | 1 |

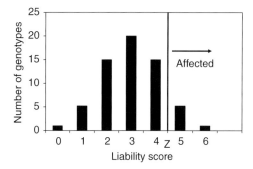

**Fig. 2.2.** Frequency distribution of genotypes by liability score under a polygenic model with three loci and threshold value Z for dichotomous traits.

M.A. Austin

### 2.3.2 Estimating heritability using twins

Twins studies are the most commonly used design to assess the heritability of a biological trait or disease. By comparing monozygous (MZ, identical) twins, who result from the division of a single zygote into two embryos and share 100% of their alleles, with dizygous (DZ, fraternal) twins who result from the fertilization of two different ova, and on average share 50% of their alleles, the proportion of the phenotypic variance attributable to genetic influences can be estimated. (Note that all MZ co-twins are the same sex, while DZ co-twins can be the same or different sexes.)

If we assume only additive genetic effects ($\sigma^2_A$) and shared equal environments for MZ and DZ co-twins in a sample, then covariances between co-twins are:

Cov (MZ) = 1.0 ($\sigma^2_A$) + 1.0 ($\sigma^2_E$) since MZ co-twins share all of their alleles, and

Cov (DZ) = 0.5 ($\sigma^2_A$) + 1.0 ($\sigma^2_E$) since DZ co-twins share half of their alleles on average.

$\sigma^2_A$ can then be estimated as:

$$2 \left[ \text{Cov (MZ)} - \text{Cov (DZ)} \right] = \left[ (\sigma^2_A + \sigma^2_E) - (0.5 (\sigma^2_A) + \sigma^2_E) \right] = \sigma^2_A$$

and heritability is:

$$h^2 = \sigma^2_A / \sigma^2_P$$

Most heritability studies based on twins use the "ACE" model, which further partitions the environmental variance into shared and non-shared components (Zuk *et al.*, 2012):

$$\sigma^2_P = \sigma^2_A + \sigma^2_C + \sigma^2_E$$

where A is due to additive genetic effects, C is due to common or shared environmental effects, and E represents a unique or non-shared environment for co-twins. Then:

$$h^2 \text{ (ACE)} = 2 (r_{MZ} - r_{DZ})$$

where r is the intraclass correlation of P between co-twins.

When $r_{MZ} > r_{DZ}$, then $h^2$ (ACE) > 0 and the trait is thought to be at least partially genetically influenced. Note that since DZ co-twins share 50% of their alleles on average, $r_{DZ}$ should also be greater than zero if genetic influences are present.

As noted above, $h^2$ can be estimated for both continuous and dichotomous traits using the polygenic model on the liability scale. Use of the ACE model to estimate genetic influences on cancer is illustrated in Box 2.2.

### 2.3.3 Assumptions, biases, and misconceptions in heritability analysis

Many assumptions are required in performing heritability analyses. When these are not met, bias in the estimates may result, possibly over- or underestimating the magnitude of genetic influences on a disease or risk factor. Further, there are a number of misconceptions about heritability. All of these concerns must be kept in mind when interpreting the results of heritability studies using twins.

### Box 2.2. Application: Heritability of Cancer

An often-cited study of genetic influences on cancer combined data from twin registries of Sweden, Denmark, and Finland to "estimate the magnitude of the genetic and
environmental effects on susceptibility to sporadic cancer" (Lichtenstein *et al.*, 2000).
These twin registries provided very large sample sizes and unique databases based
on national records.

Two birth cohorts of Swedish twins were used in the analysis, one consisting of
10,503 same-sex twins born between 1886 and 1925 who were alive in 1961. The
second cohort was 12,883 twins also of the same sex born between 1926 and
1958, who were living in 1972. Response rates for questionnaires to these twins
were 81% and 83%, respectively. Using the Swedish Mortality Registry and the
Swedish Cancer Registry, a total of 5,647 individuals were diagnosed with cancer
through 1995.

The Danish Twins Registry includes 8,461 pairs of same-sex twins born between
1870 and 1930 in which both twin pairs survived to at least age 6. Based on the Central
Register of Deaths and the Danish Cancer Registry, 3,572 individuals were diagnosed
with non-melanoma skin cancer through 1993.

The Finnish twin cohort consists of 12,941 pairs of twins living in Finland in 1975
born between 1880 and 1958. An 89% response rate was obtained for a questionnaire
sent to all twins aged 18 years or older. Twins were linked to the Finnish Cancer
Registry and the Central Population Registry and 1,584 individuals were diagnosed
with cancer through 1996.

Zygosity for all twins was obtained by questionnaire, and the ACE threshold model
was used to estimate heritability. In this context, the paper provides helpful definitions
of these components:

A: Genetic effects ($\sigma^2_A$)
  Proportion of phenotypic variance ($\sigma^2_P$) accounted for by inherited differences
  among persons
C: Shared environment ($\sigma^2_C$)
  Proportion of phenotypic variance accounted for by environmental factors shared by
  both twins
E: Non-shared environment ($\sigma^2_E$)
  Proportion of phenotypic variance accounted for by environmental factors causing
  differences between twins

The results of the heritability analysis for selected common cancers among
these twins from Nordic countries are summarized in Table 2.5. The findings show
that, for all of these cancer sites, non-shared environmental factors were the
predominant contributors to the variance in cancer, whereas shared environmental factors were generally not statistically significant. For cancer of the colorec-
tum, breast, and prostate, genetic factors explained between approximately
one-quarter and one-third of the variance. Even a decade later, with the results
of many genome-wide association studies of these cancers available, the authors'
conclusion that there are major gaps in our knowledge of genetically influenced
cancers is still valid.

*Continued*

M.A. Austin

**Box 2.2.** Continued.

**Table 2.5.** Proportion of variance explained by genetic factors, and shared and non-shared environment (adapted from Lichtenstein *et al.*, 2000).

| Cancer site | Heritability | Shared environment | Non-shared environment |
|---|---|---|---|
| Stomach | 0.28 | 0.10 | 0.62* |
| Colorectum | 0.35* | 0.05 | 0.60* |
| Pancreas | 0.36 | 0.00 | 0.64* |
| Lung | 0.26 | 0.12 | 0.62* |
| Breast | 0.27* | 0.06 | 0.67* |
| Prostate | 0.42* | 0.00 | 0.58* |

*p < 0.05

### Zygosity determination

A very basic assumption is that zygosity is accurately determined in a twin study. With new genomic technologies, zygosity determination has become more precise. However, even these techniques require the availability of DNA samples, something that may not be feasible for very large-scale studies (Forsberg *et al.*, 2010). For example, in the Scandinavian twin registries described in Box 2.2, all of the heritability estimates for cancer were based on questionnaire responses from co-twins (Sarna *et al.*, 1978). These have been documented to be accurate, but misclassification of zygosity could result in biased estimates of heritability.

### Generalizability

It is often assumed that heritability estimates based on twins are generalizable to the population at large. Although the Scandinavian twin registries are population based, the results may not be applicable to other ethnic groups or populations living in non-Nordic climates. Further, twin registries are often based on recruitment of twins from specific subpopulations (Austin *et al.*, 1987; Goldberg *et al.*, 2002). More generally, bias can be present because the magnitude of the heritability depends on the denominator, $\sigma^2_P$, which is population specific. Thus, if $\sigma^2_P$ differs among groups, there can be increases or decreases in heritability estimates, even with the same value of $\sigma^2_G$.

### Equal shared environments

As described in Section 2.3.2, another basic assumption of heritability analysis is equal shared environments for MZ and DZ co-twins. This can be expressed as:

$$\sigma^2_{E,DZ} = \sigma^2_{E,MZ}$$

---

If this assumption is true, then the estimate of the additive variance, $s^2_A$, equals the true value, $\sigma^2_A$:

$$s^2_A = 2[(\sigma^2_A + \sigma^2_{E, MZ}) - (0.5(\sigma^2_A) + \sigma^2_{E, DZ})] = \sigma^2_A$$

One might expect, however, that the environment of DZ co-twins could be less similar than for MZ co-twins, in which case:

$$\sigma^2_{E,DZ} > \sigma^2_{E,MZ} \text{ and } (\sigma^2_{E,DZ} - \sigma^2_{E,MZ}) = W > 0$$

Then:

$$s^2_A = \sigma^2_A + W > \sigma^2_A$$

and heritability can be overestimated:

$$h^2 = s^2_A / \sigma^2_P = (\sigma^2_A + W)/\sigma^2_P > \sigma^2_A / \sigma^2_P$$

In any early study based on the Kaiser-Permanente Women Twins study, we showed that environmental and behavior risk factors associated with coronary heart disease risk factors were indeed more similar among MZ co-twins compared with DZ co-twins (Austin *et al.*, 1987). For example, smoking and alcohol consumption were more similar among MZ co-twins than DZ co-twins. However, after adjusting for these factors, heritability estimates for blood pressure and body mass were not substantially altered. Thus, at least in this study, this potential source of bias did not change the interpretation of heritability estimates.

### Gene–environment interactions

Yet another assumption of heritability analysis is that there are no gene–environment interactions involved. Recently, Zuk and colleagues presented an analysis demonstrating that "heritability may be significantly inflated by genetic interactions," and introduce the concept of phantom heritability (Zuk *et al.*, 2012). They define:

$\pi_{explained}$ = proportion of $h^2$ (narrow sense) explained by a set of known genetic variants
= $h^2_{known} / h^2_{all}$

where $h^2_{known}$ = proportion of $\sigma^2_P$ explained by known additive variants and $h^2_{all}$ = proportion of $\sigma^2_P$ explained by *all* variants whether known or not.

It is generally assumed that $h^2_{all} = h^2_{pop}$

where $h^2_{pop}$ = "apparent" $h^2$ based on phenotypic correlations in the population

= $h^2_{pop}(ACE) = 2(r_{MZ} - r_{DZ})$ from twin studies

However, $h^2_{all} = h^2_{pop}$ only under a strictly additive model such as:

$$\sigma^2_P = \sigma^2_A + \sigma^2_C + \sigma^2_E$$

If there are interactions, we need to add terms to this model:

$$\sigma^2_P = \sigma^2_A + \sigma^2_C + \sigma^2_E + \sigma^2_{G*G} + \sigma^2_{G*E}$$

M.A. Austin

where $\sigma^2_{G*G}$ represents epistasis and $\sigma^2_{G*E}$ represents gene–environment interactions. In this case:

$h^2_{pop}(ACE) = h^2_{all} + W$, where $W > 0$ and thus

$h^2_{all} < h^2_{pop}$

This result shows that the heritability based on the ACE model will overestimate the heritability attributable to all genetic variants in the presence of genetic interactions. The authors coin the term phantom heritability, defined as:

$\pi_{phantom} = 1 - (h^2_{all}/h^2_{pop}) > 0$

demonstrating that even when all genetic variants contributing to a phenotype are found, there will be a "gap" between the heritability based on these variants and the population-based (ACE) estimate of heritability.

As an alternative, the authors proposed a "limited pathway" (LP) model in which a phenotype (P) depends on rate-limiting input from more than one biological pathway (Zuk et al., 2012). If K is the number of such pathways, K = 1 reduces to an additive model. As shown in Box 2.3, the LP model with K >1 can estimate heritability from observable epidemiologic parameters, including the prevalence of disease, relative risks to siblings, and $h^2_{known}$.

---

**Box 2.3. Application: Crohn's Disease**

Zuk et al. (2012) apply the LP model to Crohn's disease. Using genome-wide association studies (GWAS) and candidate gene studies, 74 different loci have been associated with risk of Crohn's disease. Based on these data, and using an additive model, $\pi_{explained} = 21.5\%$. However, under the LP(3) model that is consistent with prevalence of the disease and sib risk, $\pi_{explained} = 57.5\%$, and $\pi_{phantom} = 62.6\%$, demonstrating that the additive model of heritability appears to seriously overestimate the genetic contribution to this disease.

Overall, these findings show that the proportion of heritability explained by known genetic variants from association studies may be low because the population-based estimate of heritability is overestimated. The magnitude of this problem will be determined as new methods are developed to avoid this source of potential bias owing to gene–environment interactions.

---

## Misconceptions about heritability

Visscher and colleagues (Visscher et al., 2008) recently provided the following useful list of misconceptions about heritability, illustrating that heritability "by itself, does not provide information about the genetic architecture of the traits ...":

- $h^2$ is the proportion of phenotype passed on to the next generation.
- High $h^2$ implies genetic determination.

---

- Low $h^2$ implies no additive genetic variance.
- $h^2$ is informative about the nature of between-group differences.
- Large $h^2$ implies genes of large effect.

### Summary

As with any statistical analysis method, there are necessary assumptions and potential biases that must be considered, and the results must be interpreted correctly. This section has described several of these in relation to heritability estimates so that the reader can evaluate such analyses rigorously.

## 2.4   Conclusion: Heritability and the Polygenic Model in the Genomic Era

Although the concepts of polygenic inheritance and heritability were developed at the beginning of the 20th century, long before the current "genomic era," both ideas have taken on new relevance in the context of GWAS. As will be described in detail in Section 5.4.2, most GWAS use an additive model for single nucleotide polymorphisms (SNPs) in genetic association analyses, assuming that each susceptibility allele has an additive effect on disease susceptibility. Further, the effects sizes (ORs) in most GWAS are small, rarely exceeding 1.5, corresponding to a small effect for each susceptibility allele. These characteristics correspond closely to the polygenic model described in Section 2.3.1, and suggest that this model is a useful approach to interpreting the results from GWAS.

The concept of heritability has also been widely applied recently in estimating the proportion of genetic variance accounted for by the SNP association findings from GWAS, resulting in a lively debate about the "case of the missing heritability" (Maher, 2008; Visscher *et al.*, 2012). That is, for most diseases, genome-wide associations only explain a small proportion of the heritability as estimated from twin studies. This issue will be considered in detail in Box 5.4, using the genetics of height as an illustration.

In this chapter, we have emphasized the importance of determining the magnitude of genetic influences on diseases and risk factors as an important first step in genetic epidemiology studies. Once the extent of genetic influences has been established using familial aggregation studies and/or heritability estimates, the vast array of genomic technologies now available can be applied to identify the causal genetic variants involved and how they may interact with environmental factors to increase, or decrease, disease risk.

## Acknowledgment

The author wishes to thank Dr Bruce Weir for assistance with Section 2.3.2 of this chapter.

## Further Reading

Khoury, M.J., Beaty, T.H. and Cohen, B.H. (1993) Epidemiologic approaches to familial aggregation. In: *Fundamentals of Genetic Epidemiology*. Oxford University Press, New York, pp.164–232.

M.A. Austin

Lichtenstein, P., Holm, N.V., Verkasalo, P.K., Iliadou, A., Kaprio, J., Koskenvuo, M., *et al.* (2000) Environmental and heritable factors in the causation of cancer. Analyses of cohorts of twins from Sweden, Denmark, and Finland. *New England Journal of Medicine* 343, 78–85.

Van Dogen, J., Slagboom, P.E., Draisma, H.H.M., Martin, N.G. and Boomsma, D.I. (2012) The continuing value of twin studies in the omics era. *Nature Reviews Genetics* 13, 640–653.

Visscher, P.M., Hill, W.G. and Wray N.R. (2008) Heritability in the genomics era – concepts and misconceptions. *Nature Reviews Genetics* 9, 255–266.

# References

Amundadottir, L., Kraft, P.L., Stolzenberg-Solomon, R.Z., Fuchs, C.S., Petersen, G.M., Arslan, A.A., *et al.* (2009) Genome-wide association study identifies variants in the ABO locus associated with susceptibility to pancreatic cancer. *Nature Genetics* 41, 986–990.

Austin M.A., King M.-C., Bawol R.D., Hulley S.B. and Friedman G.D. (1987) Risk factors for coronary heart disease in adult female twins. Genetic heritability and shared environmental influences. *American Journal of Epidemiology* 125, 308–318.

Brand, R.E. and Lynch, H.T. (2006) Genotype/phenotype of familial pancreatic cancer. *Endocrinology Metabolism Clinics of North America* 35, 405–415, xi.

Breslow, N.E. and Day, N.E. (1980) Unconditional logistic regression for large strata. In: Davis, W. (ed.) *Statistical Methods in Cancer Research*. International Agency for Research on Cancer, Lyon, France, pp. 192–246.

Falconer, D.S. (1965) The inheritance of liability to certain diseases, estimated from the incidence among relatives. *Annals of Human Genetics* 29, 51–76.

Fesinmeyer, M.D., Austin, M.A., Li, C.I., De Roos, A.J. and Bowen, D.J. (2005) Differences in survival by histologic type of pancreatic cancer. *Cancer Epidemiology Biomarkers and Prevention* 14, 1766–1773.

Forsberg, C.W., Goldberg, J., Sporleder, J. and Smith, N.L. (2010) Determining zygosity in the Vietnam era twin registry: an update. *Twin Research Human Genetics* 13, 461–464.

Goldberg, J., Curran, B., Vitek, M.E., Henderson, W.G. and Boyko, E.J. (2002) The Vietnam Era Twin Registry. *Twin Research* 5, 476–481.

Jacobs, E.J., Chanock, S.J., Fuchs, C.S., Lacroix, A., McWilliams, R.R., Steplowski, E., *et al.* (2010) Family history of cancer and risk of pancreatic cancer: a pooled analysis from the Pancreatic Cancer Cohort Consortium (PanScan). *International Journal of Cancer* 127, 1421–1428.

Jones, S., Hruban, R.H., Kamiyama, M., Borges, M., Zhang, X., Parsons, D.W., *et al.* (2009) Exomic sequencing identifies *PALB2* as a pancreatic cancer susceptibility gene. *Science* 324, 217.

Khoury, M.J., Beaty, T.H. and Cohen, B.H. (1993) Epidemiologic approaches to familial aggregation. In: *Fundamentals of Genetic Epidemiology*. Oxford University Press, New York, pp.164–199.

Lichtenstein, P., Holm, N.V., Verkasalo, P.K., Iliadou, A., Kaprio, J., Koskenvuo, M., *et al.* (2000) Environmental and heritable factors in the causation of cancer. Analyses of cohorts of twins from Sweden, Denmark, and Finland. *New England Journal of Medicine* 343, 78–85.

Maher, B. (2008) The case of the missing heritability. *Nature* 456, 18–21.

Permuth-Wey, J. and Egan, K.M. (2009) Family history is a significant risk factor for pancreatic cancer: results from a systematic review and meta-analysis. *Familial Cancer* 8, 109–117.

Sarna, S., Kaprio, J., Sistonen, P. and Koskenvuo, M. (1978) Diagnosis of twin zygosity by mailed questionnaire. *Human Heredity* 28, 241–254.

Susser, E. and Susser, M. (1989) Familial aggregation studies. A note on their epidemiologic properties. *American Journal of Epidemiology* 129, 23–30.

Visscher, P.M., Hill, W.G. and Wray, N.R. (2008) Heritability in the genomics era – concepts and misconceptions. *Nature Reviews Genetics* 9, 255–266.

Visscher, P.M., Brown, M.A., McCarthy, M.I. and Yang, J. (2012) Five years of GWAS discovery. *American Journal of Human Genetics* 90, 7–24.

Wolpin, B.M., Chan, A.T., Hartge, P., Chanock, S.J., Kraft, P., Hunter, D.J., *et al.* (2009) ABO blood group and the risk of pancreatic cancer. *Journal of the National Cancer Institute* 101, 424–431.

Zuk, O., Hechter, E., Sunyaev, S.R. and Lander, E.S. (2012) The mystery of missing heritability: genetic interactions create phantom heritability. *Proceedings of the National Academy of Sciences USA* 109, 1193–1198.

# 3 Genetic Concepts and Genomic Technology for Genetic Epidemiology

MELISSA A. AUSTIN, M.S., PH.D.

*Department of Epidemiology, University of Washington, Seattle, Washington*

## Synopsis

- This chapter provides a brief review of basic concepts in human genetics and a summary of recent advances in genomic technology, with an emphasis on their relevance to genetic epidemiology.
- Concepts and topics related to single genes include: Mendelian inheritance, modes of inheritance, the Online Mendelian Inheritance in Man (OMIM®) resource, a description of the characteristics of complex genetic traits, the Hardy–Weinberg principle, the genetic code, basic gene structure, types of genetic markers including single nucleotide polymorphisms (SNPs) and copy number variants (CNVs), and the concept of identity by descent (IBD).
- Concepts and topics related to multiple genes include: genetic linkage, recombination, linkage disequilibrium, haplotypes, and tag SNPs.
- The overview of developing genomic technology describes genome-wide SNP genotyping platforms, Sanger and next-generation (massively parallel) DNA sequencing methods, and exome sequencing.
- Different study designs for investigating common and rare genetic variants are summarized.

## 3.1 Introduction

This chapter begins with a brief review of basic concepts in human genetics with an emphasis on their relevance to genetic epidemiology. It is not intended to be comprehensive, and readers are encouraged to refer to established texts (Gelehrter *et al.*, 1998; Nussbaum *et al.*, 2004; Hartl and Clark, 2007; Speicher *et al.*, 2010), especially if the genetic concepts are new. The chapter is organized to focus first on concepts related to single genes, then to principles related to multiple genes.

Next is an overview of currently available genomic technology applicable to genetic epidemiology studies. These include genome-wide SNP genotyping platforms, Sanger and next-generation (NextGen, massively parallel) DNA sequencing methods, and exome sequencing. The chapter concludes with a summary of study designs for common and rare genetic variants.

© M.A. Austin 2013. *Genetic Epidemiology: Methods and Applications*
(M.A. Austin *et al.*)

These genetic concepts and genomic technologies are essential to the research methods described in subsequent chapters, and thus are important to understand before reading those chapters.

## 3.2 Mendelian Inheritance and Complex Traits

The fact that humans are diploid and normally inherit one of each of 22 autosomal chromosomes and a sex chromosome (X or Y) from their mother and from their father means that statistical analysis for genetic epidemiology is fundamentally different from that of traditional epidemiology. That is, each participant in a study carries two alleles at any autosomal location in his or her genome. Thus, rather than the unit of analysis being an individual, each of the two alleles must be considered, and chromosomes, rather than individuals, are often the unit of analysis in genetic epidemiology. Individuals may be homozygous, carrying two identical copies of a possible disease susceptibility allele of interest; heterozygous, carrying only one of the alleles of interest; or homozygous with two identical alleles that are not thought to be associated with disease. Thus, sample size for a study can be the number of chromosomes carrying the disease susceptibility allele. In this chapter, we will use the ABO blood groups to illustrate this and other fundamental concepts of human genetics (Boxes 3.1 and 3.2).

### 3.2.1 Mendel's laws

Mendel's laws of inheritance, first described by Gregor Mendel in 1865, and subsequently rediscovered in 1900, remain fundamental to understanding genetic susceptibility to disease (Speicher *et al.*, 2010). The two laws that are most relevant to genetic epidemiology are:

- **Equal segregation:** The two alleles at a genetic locus segregate from one another and are passed to offspring with equal probability. In our example of the ABO blood groups, a parent with an AB genotype has an equal probability of passing on the A allele and the B allele to his or her offspring.

---

**Box 3.1. ABO Blood Groups**

ABO phenotypes or serotypes consist of blood group A, blood group B, and blood group O. These genetically determined blood groups were discovered in 1900 (Landsteiner, 1900) and the molecular basis of the ABO system gene on chromosome 9q34 was described in 1990 (Yamamoto *et al.*, 1990). The ABO locus encodes a glycosyltransferase with different substrate specificities and has three main variants: the A and B variants code for A and B antigens, respectively, on the surface of red blood cells, whereas O represents the lack of an antigen due to a single DNA base deletion. Thus, an individual can have one of six possible genotypes at this locus, three homozygous: AA, BB, and OO; and three heterozygous: AB, BO, and AO.

---

M.A. Austin

- **Independent assortment:** Genes on different chromosomes are inherited independently. In our example, genes located on any chromosome other than chromosome 9 (the location of the ABO locus) would be inherited independently of ABO alleles. Such genes on different chromosomes are *not* genetically "linked" to the ABO locus. Thus, in genetics, the term linkage means that two genes are close enough together on the same chromosome that they do not segregate independently.

### 3.2.2   Modes of inheritance for single genes

Phenotypes (the observed manifestation of genotypes that may be expressed physically, biochemically, or physiologically) that are inherited based on a single underlying gene depend on the mode of inheritance of that gene. These "Mendelian" traits can be:

- *Autosomal dominant:* A gene that is expressed phenotypically in both heterozygotes and homozygotes. Only one copy of a mutant allele is required for expression of the trait.
- *Recessive:* Both alleles are expressed phenotypically only in homozygotes; two copies of the mutant allele are required for expression of the trait.
- *Co-dominant or additive inheritance:* Both alleles are expressed in heterozygotes.
- *X-linked:* Genes located on the X chromosome.
- *Y-linked:* Genes located on the Y chromosome.

These modes of inheritance form the basis of segregation analysis, a statistical methodology that is used to determine whether a specific mode of inheritance is consistent with phenotypic family data, usually with the goal of identifying major gene effects on a disease of interest (Elston, 1981).

### 3.2.3   Online Mendelian Inheritance in Man (OMIM®)

The OMIM® database is a valuable resource for genetic epidemiologists, and is a "comprehensive, authoritative compendium of human genes and genetic phenotypes" (OMIM, 2012). This online catalogue is updated daily, is freely available, and provides concise reviews of all known Mendelian disorders, "with a particular focus on molecular relationship between genetic variation and phenotypic expression." It is thoroughly referenced and contains links to many other genetics resources. OMIM® is the online continuation of Dr Victor McKusick's catalog of Mendelian traits and disorders that was published in 12 book editions as *Mendelian Inheritance in Man* between 1966 and 1998. OMIM® is currently authored and edited at the Johns Hopkins School of Medicine at the McKusick–Nathans Institute of Genetic Medicine. At the time of writing, there were 21,409 entries in OMIM, 20,110 for autosomal and 1,175 for X-linked genes and phenotypes.

### 3.2.4   Complex traits

Although there are numerous clinical diseases that are caused by single-gene effects, and there has been recent emphasis on the importance of rare variants in disease susceptibility (Cirulli and Goldstein, 2010), many diseases of public health interest are common, complex traits that do not demonstrate a Mendelian mode of inheritance.

**Box 3.2. ABO Blood Group Modes of Inheritance**

In our example of ABO blood groups, A and B alleles are dominant to O, while A and B are co-dominant. The relationship between blood group (phenotype) and ABO genotype is shown in Table 3.1. Note that both AA and AO genotypes lead to A blood group phenotype, whereas only the OO genotype has an O phenotype.

These relationships are further illustrated in Fig. 3.1, in which the founder parents had genotypes AB and OO. The homozygous mother could only pass on the O allele to her offspring, while the father passed on his A allele to one son and his B allele to the second son. These sons then have genotypes AO and BO, and phenotypes A and B, respectively. The combination of dominant inheritance (A and B alleles), recessive inheritance (O allele) and co-dominant inheritance of A and B alleles is demonstrated in subsequent generations.

**Table 3.1.** Relationship between ABO genotypes and blood group phenotypes.

| ABO genotype | Blood group (phenotype) |
| --- | --- |
| AA | A |
| AO | A |
| BB | B |
| BO | B |
| AB | AB |
| OO | O |

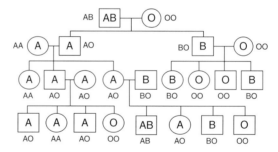

**Fig. 3.1.** Inheritance of blood groups in a hypothetical family. Blood group phenotype is shown inside each symbol and ABO genotype is shown beside or under each symbol.

Zondervan and Cardon (2004) define a complex trait as: "A measured phenotype, such as disease status or a quantitative character, which is influenced by many environmental and genetic factors, and potentially by interaction between them." Lander and Schork (1994) similarly define a complex trait to be "any phenotype that does not exhibit classic Mendelian recessive or dominant inheritance attributable to a single gene locus. … when the simple correspondence between genotype and phenotype breaks down …" They further characterize complex traits by:

- incomplete penetrance and phenocopies;
- genetic heterogeneity;

M.A. Austin

- polygenic inheritance; and
- gene–environment interactions and epistasis.

Polygenic inheritance and interactions are considered in Chapters 2 and 7, respectively, and here we define the important concepts of penetrance, phenocopy, genetic heterogeneity, and pleiotropy:

- Penetrance: The probability of expressing a phenotype given a genotype, described as either complete or incomplete and often dependent on an individual's age.
- Phenocopy: A trait that appears to be identical to a genetic trait, but that is caused by non-genetic factors.
- Genetic heterogeneity: Different genetic causes for the same disease phenotype. Although published definitions differ, two types can be distinguished:
  - Locus heterogeneity: different genes lead to the same clinical phenotype in different families.
  - Allelic heterogeneity: different alleles or mutations at the same locus results in the same clinical phenotype.
- Pleiotropy: This "occurs when one gene has an effect on multiple phenotypes" (Sivakumaran *et al.*, 2011). In an analysis of published genome-wide association studies (GWAS) from the National Human Genome Research Institute catalog, these authors recently showed that 17% of genes and 5% of genetic variants showed pleiotropic effects, indicating an important role for pleiotropy in common diseases.

## 3.3  Hardy–Weinberg Principle

The Hardy–Weinberg principle is a key concept of population genetics. It was described independently by G.H. Hardy and W. Weinberg in 1908 (Speicher *et al.*, 2010), and is an application of Mendelian genetics to populations. The Hardy–Weinberg principle explains why a dominant trait does not replace a recessive trait in the population and why allele frequencies do not change from one generation to the next in populations. Importantly for genetic epidemiology, the Hardy–Weinberg law defines the relationship between allele frequencies on chromosomes and geno-types frequencies in individuals. It is also an important assumption for genetic association studies (see Section 5.3.3).

To describe Hardy–Weinberg Equilibrium (HWE), assume that we have a single genetic locus with alleles A and a. The frequency (proportion) of allele A in the population is $f(A) = p$ (where $0 < p < 1$) and $f(a) = q$. Since A and a are the only possible alleles, $p + q = 1$ by definition. Note that, because alleles are on chromosomes, the denominators for these frequencies are the number of chromosomes carrying that allele, not the number of individuals.

If we assume that in the population of interest there is: (i) random mating; (ii) no genetic mutation; (iii) negligible migration in or out of the population; (iv) a large population size (no random drift); and (v) no natural selection operating on the locus, then it can be shown that in one generation the genotype frequencies become:

$f(AA) = p^2$

$f(Aa) = 2pq$

$f(aa) = q^2$

Further, over time, these frequencies remain the same (in equilibrium) from one generation to the next as long as the assumptions listed above prevail. The presence of HWE is equivalent to the alleles at that locus being independent from one another. As noted above, it allows the calculation of genotype frequencies from known allele frequencies. An example is shown in Box 3.3.

---

**Box 3.3. Example: Testing for Hardy–Weinberg Equilibrium**

To illustrate testing whether or not a genetic locus is in HWE, we use the example of the human chemokine receptor gene *CCR5*. It has been shown that homozygosity for a 32 bp deletion in this gene, *CCR5Δ*, confers resistance to human immunodeficiency virus infection. In a study of 338 subjects, the observed genotypes are shown in Table 3.2. Of the study subjects, 265 were homozygous for the *CCR5* wild-type genotype, while 66 were heterozygous and seven were homozygous for the deletion.

To determine whether this locus is in HWE, we must first estimate allele frequencies from the observed genotype counts, where N = number of study subjects:

p = f(*CCR5*) = [2(*CCR5*/*CCR5*) + *CCR5*/*CCR5Δ*]/2N
  = [2(265) + 66]/2(338) = 0.882

q = f(*CCR5Δ*) = [2(*CCR5Δ*/*CCR5Δ*) + *CCR5*/*CCR5Δ*]/2N = [2(7) + 66]/2(338)
  = 0.118 = 1 − p

Next, we determine expected genotype frequencies and numbers of subjects under HWE (third column of Table 3.2):

f(*CCR5*/*CCR5*) = $p^2$ = $0.882^2$ = 0.778

f(*CCR5*/*CCR5Δ*) = 2pq = 2(0.882)(0.118) = 0.208

f(*CCR5Δ*/*CCR5Δ*) = $q^2$ = (0.118) = 0.014

We multiply these frequencies by the total number of subjects to obtain the expected number of subjects with each genotype under HWE, shown in the fourth column of Table 3.2. Finally, we use a $\chi^2$ test to determine if the observed and expected numbers of subjects are statistically significantly different:

$$\chi^2 (1\,df) = \sum \frac{(Obs - Exp)^2}{Exp} = 1.42, \text{p-value} = 0.25$$

Because the p-value of 0.25 is not statistically significant, we conclude that the observed distribution of genotypes in this sample is consistent with HWE.

**Table 3.2.** Testing for HWE of gene alleles in 338 subjects (adapted from Lucotte and Mercier 1998, and Hartl and Clark, 2007).

| Genotype | Observed number of subjects | Expected frequency under HWE | Expected number of subjects under HWE |
|---|---|---|---|
| *CCR5*/*CCR5* | 265 | 0.778 | 263.0 |
| *CCR5*/*CCR5Δ* | 66 | 0.208 | 70.3 |
| *CCR5Δ*/*CCR5Δ* | 7 | 0.014 | 4.7 |

---

M.A. Austin

### 3.3.1 Deviations from Hardy–Weinberg equilibrium

In contrast to the example in Box 3.3, it is possible for genetic loci to deviate from HWE in a study. Traditionally, lack of HWE was to used evaluate whether evolutionary forces are acting on the locus of interest in the population. That is, there may be cumulative changes in the genetic composition of a population, resulting in changes in genotype and allele frequencies. These evolutionary forces include:

- Non-random mating in the population, either assortative mating or inbreeding.
- Mutation: Change in genetic material, i.e. variations in the DNA sequence.
- Natural selection: Inherited differences in the ability to survive and reproduce; over time, superior survival and reproductive genotypes increase in the population.
- Migration: movement of individuals among subpopulations.
- Random genetic drift: chance fluctuations in allele frequencies in small populations as a result of random sampling among gametes.

In the genomic era, however, departures from HWE are more often used to assess whether there are errors in the data. Specifically, departures from HWE raise the possibility of misclassification of genotypes (Weir and Laurie, 2010), and this is considered in the context of genetic association studies in Section 5.3.

## 3.4 Genetic Code, Gene Structure, and Genetic Markers

Through the processes of transcription and translation, DNA sequences of bases (A, adenine; G, guanine; C cytosine; and T, thymine) code for amino acids based on three-base triplets or "codons" that comprise the genetic code. Virtually every human genetics textbook emphasizes that the genetic code is "degenerate." That is, there are 64 such possible base triplets and only 20 amino acids (Nussbaum *et al.*, 2004). Thus, several different codons can specify the same amino acid. For example, leucine and arginine are each specified by six different codons, while tryptophan and methionine are specified by a single codon (Gelehrter *et al.*, 1998). In addition, three codons are "stop," or nonsense, codons that terminate translation of mRNA into amino acids. This "degeneracy" has important implications for genetic epidemiology because it means that there can be point mutations in the DNA sequence that change a codon, but do not change the protein encoded by a potential disease susceptibility gene. For example, if a genetic variant in a candidate gene is found to be associated with disease, but that variant does not change the protein, it can be difficult to determine if that variant is causally related to disease susceptibility.

### 3.4.1 Exons, introns, and untranslated regions

The structure and organization of a typical human gene, defined by Nussbaum *et al.* (2004) as "a sequence of chromosomal DNA that is required for production of a functional product" (including proteins) is illustrated in Fig. 3.2, from the 5′ or "upstream" end of the gene to the 3′ or "downstream" end. In addition to the exons that code for the amino acid sequence of a polypeptide chain (all exons in the human

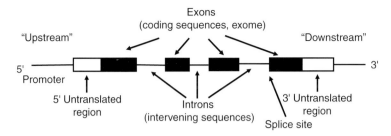

**Fig. 3.2.** General structure of a typical human gene. (Adapted from Nussbaum *et al.*, 2004.)

genome are now referred to as the "exome"), a human gene consists of: introns or intervening sequences of DNA between exons that are removed from mRNA after transcription and thus do not code for protein in translation; splice sites at junctions between introns and exons; regulatory sequences at the 5′ and 3′ ends of gene, including the promoter, DNA to which an RNA polymerase binds and initiates transcription; and 5′ and 3′ untranslated regions that are necessary for the gene expression. Many human genes are a few kilobases (kb, 1000 base pairs (bp)) long, but other genes can be hundreds of kb in length.

Because a gene contains these additional nucleotide sequences that do not code for protein, there are also polymorphisms in these regions with variants that may be linked to or associated with disease risk. In fact, in 2010, Manolio tabulated that more than 80% of variants associated with disease in GWAS are in these non-coding regions. Thus, one of the ongoing challenges in genetic epidemiology is to determine the functional significance of genomic variants associated with disease that do not change the encoded protein.

Very recently, the international Encyclopedia of DNA Elements (ENCODE) consortium published more than 30 papers as part of a large-scale project to identify all of the functional elements in the human genome sequence (Nature Encode Explorer, 2012). Among the many findings, approximately 93% of the GWAS studies to date have found diseases and traits associated with genetic variants in non-coding regions of the genome. Of these, 76% are either within or are associated with regulatory regions (Maurano *et al.*, 2012). Further, these functionally important regulatory variants may be more common in individuals than protein-coding variants, and there is also heterogeneity by cell type (Vernot *et al.*, 2012). The results of this project will continue to provide important new insights into the role of DNA variation in susceptibility to disease.

### 3.4.2 Single nucleotide polymorphisms (SNPs) and structural variations

As illustrated in Plate 1 (Altshuler *et al.*, 2008), there are many types of genetic variants in the human genome, generally referred to as "polymorphisms." In this plate, each row represents any hypothetical genetic sequence of an approximately 5 kb stretch of DNA on 20 chromosomes from ten individuals, while each column is a nucleotide. Of the 12 common variants shown, ten are common SNPs in which a single nucleotide is substituted for another nucleotide. For example, in the second column of Plate 1, 14 of the 20 chromosomes (pink and yellow) contain a C at this location, while the remaining six chromosomes contain a G. Another common variant is an insertion–deletion polymorphism ("indel") in which the same 14 chromosomes have an additional G in the sequence, while there is no such nucleotide on the remaining six chromosomes. The far right column of the figure shows a common tetranucleotide repeat variant in which the blue chromosomes have two copies of the ATTC sequence, while the purple chromosomes only have one such copy. These types of variants are also termed VNTRs for "variable number of tandem repeats." Note that, unlike SNPs, which usually have only two alleles (C and G in column 2), indels and VNTRs can have many alleles at a specific location in the genome, and thus are generally considered "more polymorphic" than SNPs.

Plate 1 also shows rare variants, including five rare SNPs designated in red (the reference nucleotides are not shown) and a larger deletion on the second to last chromosome. When these types of deletions, insertions, and/or duplications are greater than 50 bp in size, they are generally denoted CNVs or "copy number variants." Section 5.2.1 provides additional details about genetic polymorphisms in the context of candidate gene studies.

## 3.5 Genetic Linkage and Linkage Disequilibrium

### 3.5.1 Genetic linkage and recombination

In genetics, the term "linkage" has a specific and biological meaning. During meiosis and the formation of gametes, alleles on the same chromosome (linked genes) are inherited together except when crossing over (recombination) occurs during the first division of meiosis (Speicher *et al.*, 2010). First, homologous maternal and paternal chromosomes line up at the centromere during prophase I of meiosis. Crossing over, or recombination, occurs when sister chromatids on the maternal and paternal chromosomes exchange genetic material. Although this is a normal process, it breaks up associations between alleles along the same chromosome during cell division. This is illustrated in Plate 1 where a recombination "hotspot" in the genome creates little correlation between the sequence of the genome shown in pink and the sequences shown in blue and purple. The closer together two genes are on the same chromosome, the less likely recombination between them becomes. In contrast, genes on different chromosomes always segregate independently (according to Mendel's law of independent assortment), and thus are not genetically linked. This biological process is the basis of LOD score linkage analysis, as described in Section 4.1.1.

The concept of identity by descent (IBD) for a genetic marker is important for both for genetic linkage and association studies and is illustrated in Fig. 3.3. In this figure, a marker, such as a VNTR, with four alleles (a, b, c, and d) is shown to segregate in a nuclear family with five offspring. Both the parents are heterozyogtes, but with different genotypes: ab for the mother and cd for the father. The proband (arrow) inherited the a allele from the mother and the c allele from the father. His oldest sister inherited exactly the same alleles, so they share two alleles IBD. The next sister also inherited the a allele from the mother, but the d allele from the father. Thus, she shares one allele IBD (the a allele) with the proband. Similarly, the next brother with

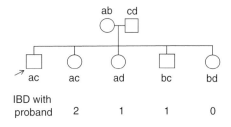

**Fig. 3.3.** Identity by descent (IBD) for a genetic marker with four alleles, a, b, c, and d.

genotype bc shares one allele IBD with the proband, but this time it is the c allele. Finally, the proband and the youngest sister with genotype bd share no alleles IBD. Depending on the degree of relationship between any two genetic relatives, the probability of sharing two, one or no alleles differs, providing the statistical basis for non-parametric linkage analysis (see Table 4.1).

### 3.5.2   Linkage disequilibrium and haplotypes

The concept of linkage disequilibrium (LD), first developed by population geneticists in the 1960s (Lewontin, 1964), is fundamental to genetic epidemiology. However, it "is one of those unfortunate terms that does not reveal its meaning" (Slatkin, 2008). LD can be defined as the non-random association, or correlation, between alleles at two loci. It is equivalent to alleles occurring on the same chromosome more (or less) often than expected from their individual allele frequencies. Returning to Plate 1, the first six nucleotides in this figure are in strong LD with each other. That is, among the pink chromosomes, every time G occurs in column 1, a C is found in column 2, T in column 3, etc. Among the yellow chromosomes, every time A is found in column 1, the same pattern is seen in columns 2 and 3, but different nucleotides are seen in columns 5 and 6. These patterns of association, or haplotypes, are common in the human genome. The International HapMap project was designed to create a genome-wide database of these patterns (Manolio *et al.*, 2008; see Section 9.3.1). The strong correlations between the first six nucleotides in the plate are indicated by red boxes below those columns, as are the blue and purple haplotypes on the right side of the figure. On either side of the recombination hotspot, however, there is little or no correlation, indicated by the white boxes.

To demonstrate how to calculate LD, consider linked genes A and B with two alleles each (Fig. 3.4). In this example, the genotyped individual is a double heterozygote with genotypes Aa and Bb at these two loci, respectively. If the capital letter alleles are on the same chromosome (Fig. 3.4a), the haplotypes are A–B and a–b. Taken together, these two haplotypes are referred to as a diplotype.

However, it is also possible that the capital letter alleles are on different chromosomes (Fig. 3.4b). In this case, the haplotypes are A–b and a–B. To determine if LD is present, we compare the frequency of haplotype A–B, f(A–B), with the allele frequencies of A and B, f(A) and f(B), in the population of interest:

If f(A–B) = f(A) × f(B), then A and B are considered to be in equilibrium. This is equivalent to alleles A and B being independent of each other.

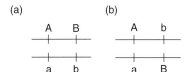

**Fig. 3.4.** Possible haplotypes of linked biallelic genes A and B.

In contrast, if $f(A–B) \neq f(A) \times f(B)$, then A and B are not independent, and disequilibrium is present. In particular, if $f(A–B) > f(A) \times f(B)$, then alleles A and B are correlated and are in LD with each other.

To calculate the magnitude of LD, we first determine the pairwise disequilibrium coefficient:

$$D = f(A–B) – f(A) \times f(B)$$

However, this is not a good measure because the possible values of D depend on the allele frequencies and D can be positive or negative. To deal with these problems, we next determine the maximum possible value of D, given the allele frequencies, that can be expressed as:

$$D_{max} = \text{Minimum } [f(A) \times f(b), f(a) \times f(B)]$$

We then standardize D using $D_{max}$ and take the absolute value:

$$D' = |D / D_{max}|$$

This measure of LD can be shown to be useful for detecting recombination between two genetic loci (Slatkin, 2008). However, for measuring correlation and for picking tag SNPs (see Section 3.5.3), another measure of LD, $r^2$, is often used:

$$r^2 = D^2/[f(A) \times f(a) \times f(B) \times f(b)]$$

Both D′ and $r^2$ range from 0, indicating little LD, to 1, indicating strong LD between alleles A and B.

For most applications of LD in genetic epidemiology, we are interested in whether known markers are in LD with a possible disease susceptibility gene, and this is illustrated in Fig. 3.5. In this setting, we are searching for a functional SNP, T, possibly in the coding region of the disease susceptibility gene. However, in most genetic linkage and association studies, we are unlikely to have genotype data on that functional SNP. Rather, we may have genotypes of surrounding SNPs, which are denoted A, B, and C in Fig. 3.5a (Zondervan and Cardon, 2004). In this hypothetical example, SNP A is located within the disease susceptibility gene, but is not the functional variant, while SNPs B and C are located outside of the gene, but are nearby on the same chromosome. For illustration, we assume that each of the markers is biallelic, with the allele frequencies shown in Table 3.3. Further, we assume that four haplotypes are observed, as shown in Fig. 3.5b. (Note that haplotype frequencies sum to one and only four of the 16 possible haplotypes are seen.)

---

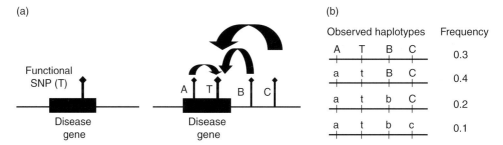

**Fig. 3.5.** (a) Unknown functional variant T in disease gene and known SNPs A, B, and C. (b) Observed haplotypes and frequencies in a hypothetical study sample for four biallelic loci, A, T, B, and C. (Adapted from Zondervan and Cardon, 2004.)

**Table 3.3.** Linkage disequilibrium between four biallelic loci (adapted from Zondervan and Cardon, 2004; see Fig. 3.5b).

| Allele frequencies | D with T | D' with T | $r^2$ with T |
|---|---|---|---|
| f(A) = 0.3, f(a) = 0.7<br>f(T) = 0.3, f(t) = 0.7 | 0.21 | 1.00 | 1.00 |
| f(B) = 0.7, f(b) = 0.3 | 0.09 | 1.00 | 0.18 |
| f(C) = 0.9, f(c) = 0.1 | 0.03 | 1.00 | 0.05 |

For example, to calculate the LD between the possible disease susceptibility loci T and marker B:

$$D = f(T–B) – f(T) \times f(B) = 0.3 – 0.3 \times 0.7 = 0.09$$

$$D_{max} = \text{minimum } [f(T) \times f(b), f(t) \times f(B)] = \text{minimum } [0.3 \times 0.3, 0.7 \times 0.7]$$
$$= \text{minimum } [0.09, 0.49] = 0.09$$

$$D' = |D/D_{max}| = 0.09/0.09 = 1.0$$

$$r^2 = D^2/[f(T) \times f(t) \times f(B) \times f(b)] = 0.09^2/[0.3 \times 0.7 \times 0.7 \times 0.3]$$
$$= 0.0081/0.0441 = 0.18$$

Thus, in this example, locus T and locus B are in "complete" LD based on D', but not based on $r^2$. This is because allele B occurs on two different haplotypes, one with allele T and another the other with allele t (Fig. 3.5b). A similar pattern is seen for the C locus. In contrast, the A allele only occurs on the haplotype with allele T. Thus, allele A is in "perfect" LD with T, with both C' and $r^2$ equal to 1.0.

Because of the many regions of high LD in the human genome, known as "haplotype blocks," most genetic epidemiology studies determine LD between all combinations of genetic markers on a particular area of interest on a chromosome. Examples will be described in Box 5.3 and Box 9.1. In addition, the size of such regions in the genome varies widely and also differs by ethnic group. For example, it has been estimated that the mean size of haplotype blocks is 22 kb in European or Asian populations, but is 11 kb among those of recent African ancestry (Manolio *et al.*, 2008).

M.A. Austin

### 3.5.3 Tag SNPs

Because of these patterns of correlation in many chromosomal regions, not all SNPs in such a region need to be genotyped for a genetic epidemiology study. Rather, a few "tag SNPs" can be selected to represent the other variants in the region. For example, as shown in Fig. 3.6, a few tag SNPs can be chosen to serve as proxies for many nucleotides (Manolio *et al.*, 2008; National Human Genome Research Institute, 2008).

In this example, a sequence of 32 nucleotides is shown for six chromosomes (Fig. 3.6a). First, note that there is no variation in 24 of the 32 nucleotides, shown in grey. Assuming that these six chromosomes represent most of the haplotypes in this region of the genome in the population of interest, these 24 nucleotides are not informative for genetic epidemiology studies, and thus do not need to be genotyped. Next, in block 1, there are four SNPs. However, these SNPs are in perfect LD. That is, every time an A occurs in SNP1, there is a C for SNP2, a G for SNP3, and an A for SNP4. Thus, the information in these four SNPs is completely redundant, and genotyping one SNP, in this case SNP3, completely characterizes the variation in this block. Similarly for block 2, every time a G is present for SNP5, a T is present for SNP6 and an A is present for SNP7. Thus, only SNP6 needs to be genotyped. Finally, SNP8 is a "singleton" in that it is not correlated with any of the other SNPs, and provides additional information on genomic variation. Taken together, genotyping three SNPs provides all of the available data for these 32 nucleotides (Fig. 3.6b). In addition to the pattern of LD in a genomic region, the selection of tag SNPs is also based on the technical ease of genotyping, which can vary among genetic markers.

Similar to the situation shown in Fig. 3.5a, tag SNPs are especially useful when searching for an unknown functional disease susceptibility allele that may not be genotyped. This approach was first developed for candidate gene studies (Carlson *et al.*, 2004), and is now extensively used for GWAS. This type of "indirect association" is described further in Section 5.3.2.

### 3.5.4 SNP genotyping platforms

Using information generated by the HapMap project on more than 3 million SNPs in the human genome, the initial set of SNP genotyping platforms was

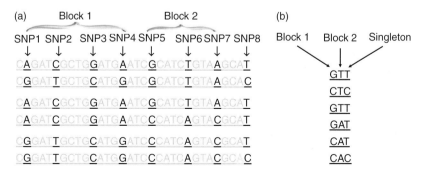

**Fig. 3.6.** (a) Eight SNPs within a sequence of 32 nucleotides from six chromosomes. (b) Three tag SNPs serve as proxies for 32 nucleotides. (Adapted from National Human Genome Research Institute, 2008.)

---

**Table 3.4.** Comparison of estimated coverage for commercially available genome-wide SNP genotyping platforms (adapted from Manolio *et al.*, 2008; National Human Genome Research Institute, 2008).

| | Percentage of SNPs tagged at $r^2 \geq 0.8$ | | |
|---|---|---|---|
| Genotyping platform | HapMap Yoruba sample in Ibadan, Nigeria (YRI) | HapMap subsample of Utah residents of northern European descent (CEU) | HapMap Han Chinese in Beijing and Japanese in Tokyo (CHB + JPT) |
| Affymetrix GeneChip 500K | 46 | 68 | 67 |
| Affymetrix SNP Array 6.0 | 66 | 82 | 81 |
| Illumina HumanHap300 | 33 | 77 | 63 |
| Illumina HumanHap550 | 55 | 88 | 83 |
| Illumina HumanHap650Y | 66 | 89 | 84 |
| Perlegen 600K | 47 | 92 | 84 |

developed by taking advantage of LD in the human genome. These arrays made GWAS possible (Manolio *et al.*, 2008). As shown in Table 3.4, the coverage of the genome by these platforms differed by ethnic group. As expected, populations such as those of African descent have less coverage than European populations because of lower LD. However, as genotyping technology has developed, this coverage has improved dramatically. In fact, because of smaller haplotype blocks and differences in allele frequencies in non-European ethnic groups, these populations can be particularly suitable for localizing a functional disease variant once its chromosomal region has been identified (Reiner *et al.*, 2012). This is because the distance between the tag SNPs and the causal variant may be smaller in such populations (Rosenberg *et al.*, 2010).

More recent examples of arrays for genotyping include the Affymetrix Genome-Wide Human SNP Array 6.0, which contains 906,000 SNPs: 482,600 SNPs from previous arrays based on HapMap and diversity panels, and an additional 424,000 SNPs that include tag SNPs, SNPs from the X and Y chromosomes, mitochondrial SNPs, new SNPs from the HapMap database, and SNPs in recombination hotspots; and Illumina, Inc. arrays such as the Omni V chip that use the Bead Chip Infinium Technology (Institute of Translational Health Sciences, 2011).

## 3.6 DNA Sequencing Technologies

In contrast to genome-wide SNP chips that are designed primarily to detect common variation, DNA sequencing, including exome sequencing, can detect rare genetic variants. This is important for complex diseases, as well as Mendelian diseases, because functionally deleterious variants are expected to be present in most genes, although they may be rare. Currently, this is an extremely active area of research and several applications of DNA sequencing to genetic epidemiology are described in subsequent chapters.

M.A. Austin

### 3.6.1  Three generations of DNA sequencing

"First-generation" automated Sanger sequencing, designed to read the sequence of base pairs in a region of DNA, was introduced in 1977 (Sanger *et al.*, 1977). It was used to obtain the first entire sequence of a human genome for the Human Genome Project in 2001 (Lander *et al.*, 2001; Venter *et al.*, 2001). Although sequencing platforms have evolved rapidly since that time, Sanger sequencing remains the "gold standard" for clinical sequencing, including for cytogenetics. This is because it is still the most accurate method for sequencing, with an average of <1% error rate, and it has a well-defined chemistry (Rizzo and Buck, 2012). The process of DNA sequencing involves four steps (Institute of Translational Health Sciences, 2011):

1. Generation of a nested set of DNA fragments using chemical or enzymatic methods.
2. Separation of the fragments using electrophoretic methods.
3. Detection of bases using labeling chemistries with four-color fluorescent dyes.
4. Analysis or base calling.

Applications of Sanger sequencing are now restricted owing to limitations of its cost and "throughput," that is, the amount of DNA sequence that can be read with each reaction. Specifically, each Sanger instrument can only read 96 reactions in parallel, with read lengths of 500 bp to 1 kb, and run times limit the throughput per day (Rizzo and Buck, 2012). In addition, this method requires a relatively large amount of DNA, and often needs other methods such as physical mapping for ordering DNA clones before sequencing of the nested fragments (Institute of Translational Health Sciences, 2011).

In contrast, "next-generation" (NextGen) or "massively parallel" DNA sequencing allows hundreds of millions of reads at a much lower cost. These high-throughput technologies "are capable of sequencing large numbers of different DNA sequences in a single reaction" (Rizzo and Buck, 2012), hence the term "parallel," and most use dye-labeled modified nucleotides (Metzker, 2010). The trade-off is that NextGen sequencing has short read lengths (30–400 bp) and lower sequence quality. The common element of these methods is that they "monitor the sequential addition of nucleotides to immobilized and spatially arrayed DNA templates" (Rizzo and Buck, 2012).

Within NextGen sequencing technologies, "second-generation" methods use amplification-based approaches. That is, following sample collection, the steps involved in such sequencing experiments for either human whole-genome resequencing or exome sequencing are (Metzker, 2010; Rizzo and Buck, 2012):

1. Sequencing library/template generation: Create an unbiased sequencing library that is representative of the DNA sample. This involves fragmentation, the creation of smaller DNA fragments that can be sequenced.
2. Sequencing and imaging: Methods include sequencing by synthesis, reversible dye terminators, and sequencing by ligation (Institute of Translational Health Sciences, 2011).
3. Data analysis: After base calling, the sequencing data are either aligned to a known reference sequence or are assembled *de novo*.

It is important to take note of the potential sources of bias and error in second-generation sequencing. These include the following:

- Sequencing errors can be created during template amplification by introducing mutations that may later appear to be sequence variants.
- Because of short read lengths, repetitive regions of the genome may not be aligned to the reference genome uniquely, and structural variations (insertions, deletions, translocations) can be challenging to align.
- "Coverage or depth": the average number of times a particular DNA base pair is sequenced in a particular experiment can be non-uniform and biased, possibly leaving portions of the genome undersequenced or even unsequenced, and precluding the identification of SNPs and structural variants. "Deep coverage" of 80× or 100× avoids errors, but has the trade-off of reducing the number of samples that can be sequenced, and thus limiting the ability to detect rare variants.
- Quality and quantity of sample DNA need to be optimized for the specific platform being used.
- Accuracy of base calling rates can differ such that the initial portion of each sequence read is typically more accurate than the later reads due to signal decay.

The "third generation" of DNA sequencing technologies are referred to as "single molecule systems." Unlike second-generation approaches, they do not require amplification steps, avoiding potential errors, can be used to sequence very small quantities of DNA, and will likely provide longer read lengths (Rizzo and Buck, 2012). At least three different methodologies are now entering the market (Institute of Translational Health Sciences, 2011).

Ongoing advances in all of these methods continue to rapidly increase throughput, decrease the expense of DNA sequencing, and improve accuracy. For example, a new method, "duplex sequencing," has recently been developed that reduces errors by sequencing both strands of DNA (Schmitt *et al.*, 2012). However, these developments are also creating a widening gap between the cost of actually generating the data and the cost of data analysis and interpretation, storing megabases (millions) to gigabases (billions) of data points, and quality control of this high volume of data (Institute of Translational Health Sciences, 2011; Rizzo and Buck, 2012). These challenges will need to be met by continuing advances in bioinformatics. Further, even with plummeting costs, whole-genome sequencing for humans is still expensive. Thus, current approaches, including exome sequencing, that target or are enriched for specific areas of interest in the genome are the most feasible for genetic epidemiology studies at this time.

### 3.6.2   Exome sequencing

The exome, the subset of the genome that is protein coding, consists of approximately 180,000 exons and about 30 megabases of sequence. It constitutes less than 2% of the genome, includes splice sites and micro RNAs, but does not include

5' or 3' untranslated regions. The number of exons per gene varies considerably, but most genes have between one and ten exons. Advantages of sequencing the exome, rather than the whole genome, are that it requires much less sequencing, and that variants in exomes are likely to have larger-sized effects on traits because they disrupt the protein-coding sequences and are more interpretable because they are likely to have functional consequences. The major disadvantage of exome sequencing is that it misses non-coding variants that may influence disease risk.

As described by Bamshad *et al.* (2011), the basic steps required for exome sequencing are as follows:

1. Genomic DNA is randomly sheared and used to construct a "shotgun" library of fragments.
2. The library is enriched for sequences corresponding to exons and these fragments are hybridized to DNA or RNA baits.
3. Recovery of hybridized fragments.
4. Massively parallel sequencing of the enriched, amplified library.
5. Mapping, alignment, and variant calling.

Rigorous quality control of exome sequencing data procedures is essential to avoid distorting association results. Ongoing challenges include (Metzker, 2010; Bamshad *et al.*, 2011; Kiezun *et al.*, 2012) the following:

- Several micrograms of high-quality DNA are needed as starting material.
- Defining and "capturing" the exome within the genome is challenging because there is still uncertainty about which genome sequences are truly protein-coding and the efficiency of capture probes varies, and not all sequences can be aligned to the reference genome. Because of variation in capture technologies, cases and controls should always be processed using the same technology to avoid differential detection of variants among batches.
- There is a high degree of variability coverage of the exome, with portions of the exome poorly covered or completely missed.
- Detecting small indels and copy number changes from short-read exome sequence data needs improvement. Some regions may be over-covered or under-covered due to technical artifacts rather than representing true structural variation.
- Importantly, causal variants can be difficult to identify among the more than 20,000 single nucleotide variants often identified from the exome sequence of a given sample (Ng *et al.*, 2010). That is, distinguishing between background polymorphisms and possible disease-causing mutations using filtering is essential for high-quality variant calls. Several filtering approaches can be used, including identifying causal mutations based on function (missense, nonsense, coding indels, and splice sites in coding regions), ranking variants by their effect on protein structure and conservation scores based on software tools such as SIFT and PolyPhen (Ng *et al.*, 2010).

Methods for statistical analysis of data from DNA sequencing studies, including exome sequencing, are described in Section 5.8.

## 3.7 Study Designs for Common and Rare Genetic Variants

The frequency of potential disease-causing genetic variants is one important element in deciding the study design to use for a genetic epidemiology study. Depending on the frequency of the less common allele at a locus, the "minor allele frequency," different analysis approaches are applicable (Table 3.5), all of which will be considered in subsequent chapters. In particular, as genomic technology has rapidly progressed, including advancing from genome-wide SNP arrays for detecting common variants to detecting rare alleles using sequencing, a variety of study designs can now be considered for mapping disease susceptibility loci. For example, as discussed in Section 5.8, methods for discovering association of rare genetic variants with disease risk are different from those used for association with common genetic variants because rare variants must be combined in a gene, a biological pathway, or a regulatory region rather than testing for common individual variants.

## 3.8 Conclusion

Understanding both the fundamental concepts of human genetics and being aware of the recent technological advances in genomics are essential for developing successful genetic epidemiology research projects. This chapter has provided a summary of these as the basis for subsequent chapters describing genetic epidemiology research methods and their applications.

**Table 3.5.** Minor allele frequencies, class of genetic variants, and analysis approaches (adapted from Cirulli and Goldstein, 2010).

| Minor allele frequency | Class of variant | Analysis approaches |
|---|---|---|
| 5–50% | Very common | Genome-wide association studies (see Section 5.4) |
| 1–5% | Less common | Association analysis using variants from 1000 Genomes Project (see Section 9.3.2) |
| Less than 1%, but still polymorphic in the population | Rare | Exome sequencing, sequencing affected relatives in families, or extreme trait sequencing (see Box 4.3 and Section 5.8) |
| Only present in affected probands and relatives | Private | Co-segregation (linkage) in affected families (see Section 4.1) |

M.A. Austin

## Acknowledgments

The author would like to thank Dr. Susan Heckbert for content in Section 3.5, and Dr. Deborah A. Nickerson, Dr. Roger Bumgarner, and the University of Washington Institute of Translation Health Sciences (UL1TR000423) for material in Section 3.6.

## Further Reading

Altschuler, D., Daly, M.J. and Lander, E.S. (2008) Genetic mapping in human disease. *Science* 322, 881–888.

Gelehrter, T.D., Collins, F.S. and Ginsberg, D. (1998) *Principles of Medical Genetics*, 2nd edn. William & Wilkins, Baltimore, Maryland.

Green, E.D., Guyer, M.S. and National Human Genome Research Institute (2011) Charting a course for genomic medicine from base pairs to bedside. *Nature* 470, 204–213.

Hartl, D.L. and Clark, A.G. (2007) *Principles of Population Genetics*, 4th edn. Sinauer Associates, Inc., Sunderland, Massachusetts.

Speicher, M.R., Antonarakis, S.E. and Motulsky, A.G. (2010) *Vogel and Motulsky's Human Genetics. Problems and Approaches*, 4th edn. Springer-Verlag, Berlin.

## References

Altschuler, D., Daly, M.J. and Lander, E.S. (2008) Genetic mapping in human disease. *Science* 322, 881–888.

Bamshad, M.J., Ng, S.B., Bigham, A.W., Tabor, H.K., Emond, M.J., Nickerson, D.A. and Shendure, J. (2011) Exome sequencing as a tool for Mendelian disease gene discovery. *Nature Reviews Genetics* 12, 745–755.

Carlson, C.S., Eberle, M.A., Rieder, M.J., Yi, Q., Kruglyak, L. and Nickerson, D.A. (2004) Selecting a maximally informative set of single-nucleotide polymorphisms for association analyses using linkage disequilibrium. *American Journal of Human Genetics* 74, 106–120.

Cirulli, E.T. and Goldstein, D.B. (2010) Uncovering the roles of rare variants in common disease through whole-genome sequencing. *Nature Reviews Genetics* 11, 415–425.

Elston, R.C. (1981) Segregation analysis. *Advances in Human Genetics* 11, 63–120.

Gelehrter, T.D., Collins, F.S. and Ginsberg, D. (1998) *Principles of Medical Genetics*, 2nd Edn. William & Wilkins, Baltimore, Maryland.

Hartl, D.L. and Clark, A.G. (2007) *Principles of Population Genetics*, 4th Edn. Sinauer Associates, Inc., Sunderland, Massachusetts.

Institute of Translational Health Sciences (ITHS), University of Washington (2011) A Short Course on DNA Analysis Technologies. Available from: https//www.iths.org/events/short-course-dna-analysis-technologies (accessed September 12, 2012).

Kiezun, A., Garilmella, K., Do, R., Stitziel, N.O., Neale, B.M., McLaren P.J., *et al.* (2012) Exome sequencing and the genetic basis of complex traits. *Nature Genetics* 44, 623–629.

Lander, E.S. and Schork, N.J. (1994) Genetic dissection of complex traits. *Science* 265, 2037–2048.

Lander, E.S., Linton, L.M., Birren, B., Nusbaum, C., Zody, M.C., Baldwin, J., *et al.* (2001) Initial sequencing and analysis of the human genome. *Nature* 409, 860–921.

Landsteiner, K. (1900) Zur Kenntnis der antifermentativen, lytischen und agglutinierenden Wirkungen des Blutserums und der Lymphe. *Zentralblatt Bakteriologie* 27, 357–362.

Lewontin, R.C. (1964) The interaction of selection and linkage. I. General considerations; heterotic model. *Genetics* 49, 49–67.

Lucotte, G. and Mercier, G. (1998) Distribution of CCR5 gene 32-bp deletion in Europe. *Journal of Acquired Immune Deficiency Syndromes and Human Retrovirology* 19, 174–177.

Manolio, T.A. (2010) Genomewide association studies and assessment of the risk of disease. *New England Journal of Medicine* 363, 166–176.

Manolio, T.A., Brooks, L.D. and Collins, F.S. (2008) A HapMap harvest of insights into the genetics of common disease. *Journal of Clinical Investigation* 118, 1590–1605.

Maurano, M.T., Humbert, R., Rynes, E., Thurman, R.E., Haugen, E., Wang, H., *et al.* (2012) Systematic localization of common disease-associated variation in regulatory DNA. *Science* 337, 1190–1195.

Metzker, M.L. (2010) Sequencing technologies – the next generation. *Nature Reviews Genetics* 11, 31–46.

National Human Genome Research Institute (2008) Genetics for Epidemiologists: Application of Human Genomics to Population Sciences. Available from: http://www.genome.gov/27026645 (accessed September 13, 2012).

Nature Encode Explorer (2012) Available from: www.nature.com/encode (accessed November 26, 2012).

Ng, S.B., Nickerson, D.A., Bamshad, M.J. and Shendure, J. (2010) Massively parallel sequencing and rare disease. *Human Molecular Genetics* 19, R119–R124.

Nussbaum, R.L., McInnes, R.R. and Willard, H.F. (2004) *Thompson & Thompson Genetics in Medicine*, 6th edn, Revised Reprint. Saunders, an imprint of Elsevier, Philadelphia, Pennsylvania, pp. 20–21.

OMIM (Online Mendelian Inheritance in Man®) (2012) Available from: http://www.omim.org/ (accessed September 17, 2012).

Reiner, A.P., Beleza, S., Franceschini, N, Auer, P.L., Robinson, J.G. and Kooperbert, C. *et al.* (2012) Genome-wide association and population genetic analysis of C-reactive protein in African American and Hispanic American women. *American Journal of Human Genetics* 91, 502–512.

Rizzo, J.M. and Buck, M.J. (2012) Key principles and clinical applications of "next-generation" DNA sequencing. *Cancer Prevention Research* 5, 887–900.

Rosenberg, N.A., Huang, L., Jewett, E.M., Szpiech, Z.A., Jankovic, I. and Boehnke, M (2010) Genome-wide association studies in diverse populations. *Nature Reviews Genetics* 11, 356–366.

Sanger, F., Nicklen, S. and Coulson, A.R. (1977) DNA sequencing with chain-terminating inhibitors. *Proceedings of the National Academy of Sciences USA* 74, 5463–5467.

Schmitt, M.W., Kennedy, S.R., Salk, J.J., Fox, E.J., Hiatt, J.B. and Loeb, L.A. (2012) Detection of ultra-rare mutations by next-generation sequencing. *Proceedings of the National Academy of Sciences USA* 109, 14508–14513.

Sivakumaran, S., Agakov, F., Theodoratou, E., Prendergast, J.G., Zgaga, L., Manolio, T., *et al.* (2011) Abundant pleiotropy in human complex diseases and traits. *American Journal of Human Genetics* 89, 607–618.

Slatkin, M. (2008) Linkage disequilibrium – understanding the evolutionary past and mapping the medical future. *Nature Reviews Genetics* 9, 477–485.

Speicher, M.R., Antonarakis, S.E. and Motulsky, A.G. (2010) *Vogel and Motulsky's Human Genetics. Problems and Approaches*, 4th edn, Springer-Verlag, Berlin.

Venter, J.C., Adams, M.D., Myers, E.W., Li, P.W., Mural, R.J. Sutton, G.G., *et al.* (2001) The sequence of the human genome. *Science* 291, 1304–1351.

Vernot, B., Stergachis, A.B., Maurano, M.T., Vierstra, J., Neph, S., Thurman, R.E., *et al.* (2012) Personal and population genomics of human regulatory variation. *Genome Research* 22, 1689–1697.

M.A. Austin

Weir, B.S. and Laurie, C.C. (2010) Characterizing allelic association in the genome era. *Genetics Research Cambridge* 92, 461–470.

Yamamoto, F., Clausen, H., White, T., Marken, J. and Hakomori, S. (1990) Molecular genetic basis of the histo-blood group ABO system. *Nature* 345, 229–233.

Zondervan, K.T. and Cardon, L.R. (2004) The complex interplay among factors that influence allelic association. *Nature Reviews Genetics* 5, 89–100.

# 4 Family Studies in Genetic Epidemiology: From Linkage to Exome Sequencing

MELISSA A. AUSTIN, M.S., PH.D.,[1]
TERRI H. BEATY, PH.D.,[2] AND
JANET L. STANFORD, M.P.H., PH.D.[3]

[1]*Department of Epidemiology, University of Washington, Seattle, Washington;* [2]*Department of Epidemiology, Johns Hopkins University, Baltimore, Maryland;* [3]*Division of Public Health Sciences, Fred Hutchinson Cancer Research Center, Department of Epidemiology, University of Washington, Seattle, Washington*

## Synopsis

- Family studies remain a fundamental component of genetic epidemiology for discovering disease susceptibility genes.
- LOD score linkage analysis compares the number of recombinant and non-recombinant offspring to search for evidence of co-segregation between a hypothetical disease gene and a known genetic marker.
- Non-parametric linkage analysis uses excess sharing of marker alleles identical by descent (IBD), especially siblings, for a linkage analysis approach in the absence of multi-generational family data.
- Genetic association studies can also be conducted in families, often using parent–offspring trios.
- Over the last two decades, family studies in genetic epidemiology have evolved from using linkage analysis to exome sequencing for finding disease susceptibility genes, providing major progress in our understanding of genetic susceptibility to both rare, familial forms of disease, and common, complex diseases.
- These advances are illustrated with examples from research on familial breast cancer, familial pancreatic cancer, and familial prostate cancer.
- The goal of all of these research approaches is to use molecular discoveries to better diagnose, treat, and prevent disease.

## 4.1 Linkage Analysis

### 4.1.1 Basics of LOD score linkage analysis

LOD score linkage analysis, one of the fundamental approaches for mapping disease genes, is based on searching for evidence of co-segregation of disease with known

© M.A. Austin 2013. *Genetic Epidemiology: Methods and Applications*
(M.A. Austin *et al.*)

genetic markers within families (Khoury *et al.*, 1993). The goal of linkage analysis is to identify the approximate chromosomal location of a disease susceptibility gene.

The biological basis, and thus the interpretation of linkage analysis, is straightforward. During meiosis and the formation of gametes, alleles on the same chromosome (linked genes) are inherited together except when crossing over (recombination) occurs during the first division of meiosis. First, homologous maternal and paternal chromosomes line up at the centromere during prophase I of meiosis. Crossing over, or recombination, occurs when sister chromatids on the maternal and paternal chromosomes exchange genetic material. Although this is a normal process, it breaks up associations between alleles along the same chromosome during cell division. Further, the closer together two genes are on the same chromosome, the less likely recombination between them becomes. In contrast, genes on different chromosomes always segregate independently (according to Mendel's law of independent assortment), and thus are not genetically linked. As a result, the frequency of crossing over depends on the physical distance between two syntenic genes, and this creates a means to identify deviation from independent segregation and to estimate the genetic distance between two genes. Comparing this null hypothesis of no linkage (independent assortment or 50% recombination) with the alternative hypothesis of linkage (where recombination is reduced) gives a statistical test for linkage and allows the genetic distance (in terms of recombination rate) to be estimated. This same approach can be used to show evidence of co-segregation between an observed marker and a hypothetical gene controlling a disease phenotype, which provides evidence of linkage to map a previously unknown causal gene. Because linkage is based on the physical distance between two genes, it is a property of loci along a chromosome, not the alleles at these loci.

How linkage analysis is used for mapping disease genes is illustrated in Fig. 4.1. In this family, we assume there is a dominant mode of inheritance for a relatively rare Mendelian disease with full penetrance (shown as filled in symbols). The grandmother in this family appears to pass on the disease gene to her son along with the solid black chromosome. Similarly, her son in generation 2 appears to have passed on the causal mutation in the disease gene to the first grandson in generation 3 with the same solid black chromosome completely intact. The affected granddaughter in generation 3, however, only inherited the bottom two-thirds of this chromosome because of recombination during meiosis in her father, so she is termed a "recombinant" offspring. This particular family provides evidence that the disease gene is located on this

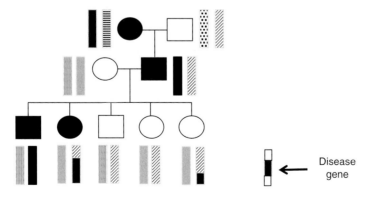

**Fig. 4.1.** Example of linkage analysis in a three-generation family for a dominant disease with full penetrance. Chromosomes are shown as patterned rectangles.

lower portion of the checkerboard chromosome. The next grandson and grand-daughter did not inherit the disease mutation or the solid black chromosome, having received the grandpaternal chromosome from their father. Finally, the youngest granddaughter did not inherit the disease mutation from her father although she did receive part of the grandmaternal chromosome (just not the part carrying the causal mutation), and is also a recombinant. Due to recombination, this last child did inherit the bottom one-quarter of the solid black chromosome, suggesting the disease muta-tion is not in this segment of the solid black chromosome. Taken together, these data provide evidence the causal gene may be located somewhere in the middle of the solid black chromosome. Of course, this is only one family, and more families would be needed to definitively map the chromosomal location of this disease gene.

As described below, the parameter θ (defined as the probability (P) of observing a recombinant gamete) is used in linkage analysis to quantify recombination between two loci (two markers or one marker and a causal gene controlling a disease) in LOD score linkage analysis. Figure 4.2 illustrates sister chromatids from homologous chromosomes lined up in the first division of meiosis. In Fig. 4.2a, genes A and B are closely linked on the long arm of the chromosome, and this individual is heterozygous at both of these loci (the person's genotype is Aa and Bb). Because recombination is unlikely during meiosis in this setting, the only observed gametes from meiosis I are A–B and a–b. When there are no such recombinant gametes, θ = P(observing a recombinant gamete) = 0, which is termed complete linkage. In Fig. 4.2b, genes A and B are both still on the long arm of the chromo-some, but they are far apart. Thus, it is more likely recombination will take place during meiosis I, resulting in both non-recombinant gametes (A–B and a–b) and recombinant gametes (A–b and a–B). In this situation, θ = P(observing a recombinant gamete) > 0. Finally, in Fig. 4.3, genes A and B are not linked, and are on different chromosomes. In this situation, both apparent non-recombinant (A–B and a–b) and recombinant (A–b and a–B) gametes are all equally possible under Mendel's law of independent assortment, and θ = P (observing a recombinant gamete) = ½. Therefore, θ ranges from 0 (complete linkage) to ½ (no linkage), and values in between 0 and ½ indicate possible linkage of genes A and B.

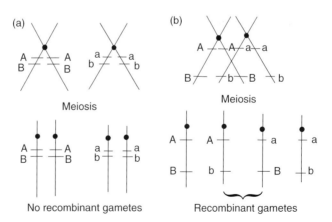

**Fig. 4.2.** Illustration of sister chromatids from a homologous pair of chromosomes, locations of linked genes A and B, and gametes resulting from meiosis. (a) Closely linked genes on the long arm of the same chromosome. (b) Crossing over occurs between genes A and B during meiosis.

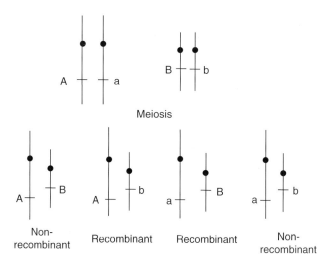

**Fig. 4.3.** Illustration of two homologous pairs of chromosomes, locations of unlinked genes A and B, and gametes resulting from meiosis.

LOD scores are statistics used to evaluate linkage between a known genetic marker and a potential disease gene under investigation, and are based on unscaled likelihood functions $L(\theta)$ that are proportional to probabilities:

$L(\theta)$ = likelihood ($\theta$ | family data) $\propto$ P(family data | $\theta$).

We need to calculate the likelihood of observing the co-segregation of a causal disease allele and the observed markers, such as illustrated in Fig. 4.1, given some specified value of $\theta$ between 0 and ½. We then want to compare this likelihood function $L(\theta)$ for the case of linkage, i.e. when $\theta < ½$, with $L(\theta)$ to no linkage, i.e. when $\theta = ½$. This is accomplished by taking the ratio of these two likelihoods, or the odds ratio (OR):

$OR = L(\theta < ½)/L(\theta = ½)$

If this OR > 1, there is evidence for linkage in the family, whereas if OR < 1, the data gives evidence against linkage. We can then take the $\log_{10}$ of this OR, which is termed the LOD score, or Z score:

$LOD(\theta) = \log_{10}(L(\theta)/L(½)) = \log_{10}(OR) = Z(\theta)$

This calculation is performed for each family independently in the linkage analysis, and the Z scores are summed for all families (the equivalent of multiplying likelihoods). If we define $Z_i(\theta)$ to be the LOD score for family i of i = 1,...n families in a study, then the overall LOD score becomes the sum of the LOD scores for all families:

$Z(\theta) = \Sigma Z_i(\theta)$ for i = 1,...n

An overall Z score of +3 corresponds to an OR of $10^3$ or 1000:1 odds in favor of linkage, whereas an LOD score of –2 corresponds to an OR of $10^{-2}$ or 100:1 odds against linkage. These threshold values of +3 and –2 are traditionally used to declare statistically significant evidence at the $\alpha = 0.05$ level, for linkage and lack of linkage, respectively.

---

In summary, LOD score linkage analysis makes use of independent families where recombinant and non-recombinant offspring are counted to search for evidence of co-segregation between a hypothetical disease gene and a known genetic marker. Linkage analysis is unique because there is a solid biological basis behind these statistics, i.e. crossing over during meiosis. Linkage analysis involves estimating the genetic recombination fractions, and testing hypotheses about linkage versus no linkage is based on LOD scores. This approach has been in use for many years, and works best for rare, Mendelian disorders (Ott *et al.*, 2011), as illustrated by the applications in Boxes 4.1 and 4.3. Readers who are interested in more advanced linkage analysis methods, including multipoint mapping for analysis of more than two loci at a time, are encouraged to refer to Khoury *et al.* (1993) and Ott (1999).

### 4.1.2 Non-parametric linkage analysis

LOD score linkage analysis requires multiplex families (where >1 member is affected) and can only be fully informative when one parent is a double heterozygote (AaBb) because this allows all children to be classified as recombinant or non-recombinant without ambiguity. Multi-generation families with many children are more informative for linkage studies than smaller, nuclear families (parents and their children). Larger, multi-generation families with many offspring from informative parents can provide definitive evidence of linkage for rare, Mendelian traits, although there is always a lower limit to the resolution in linkage analysis (generally 5–10 centiMorgans or approximately 5–10 megabases of physical distance) due to the limited number of informative meiotic events available. Also, such large multiplex families are highly unusual and difficult to ascertain, so alternative study designs have been developed to test for the effects of linkage using nuclear families with ≥2 affected siblings. This non-parametric linkage analysis tests for a consequence of linkage rather than trying to estimate $\theta$ directly and test the null hypothesis of no linkage ($\theta = \frac{1}{2}$) by focusing on testing for excess sharing of marker alleles that are identical by descent (IBD, see Chapter 3) between full siblings selected because of their phenotype (i.e. pairs or sets of siblings ascertained because they were affected with disease).

All biological relatives have a fixed prior probability of sharing 0, 1, or 2 alleles IBD at any autosomal gene based solely on their relationship. Table 4.1 lists these probabilities for several common relationships. If we selectively sample sets of affected relatives

**Table 4.1.** Prior probability of sharing 0, 1, or 2 alleles IBD for different types of relative pairs.

| Relative pair | Degree (°) of relationship | Alleles shared IBD | | |
|---|---|---|---|---|
| | | 2 | 1 | 0 |
| Parent–offspring | 1° | 0.0 | 1.0 | 0.0 |
| Full siblings | 1° | 0.25 | 0.5 | 0.25 |
| Half siblings | 2° | 0.0 | 0.5 | 0.5 |
| Grandparent–grandchild | 2° | 0.0 | 0.5 | 0.5 |
| Avuncular | 2° | 0.0 | 0.5 | 0.5 |
| First cousins | 3° | 0.0 | 0.25 | 0.75 |
| Monozygous twins[a] | 0° | 1 | 0 | 0 |

[a]Bilineal relationship.

M.A. Austin *et al.*

(e.g. pairs of affected siblings), we can then test for excess allele sharing in these selected samples. If a marker is truly not linked to a gene influencing risk, the observed pattern of IBD sharing should not deviate from expected, but if the marker is linked to such a causal gene there should be excess IBD sharing between affected full siblings. This approach is termed non-parametric linkage, because it does not involve estimating any parameter (such as the recombination fraction) but rather merely tests for adherence to the prior probabilities. Rejecting the null hypothesis constitutes evidence of excess allele sharing, which would result from linkage between an observed marker and an unobserved causal gene. Because non-parametric linkage is most often based on affected sibling pairs, collecting families becomes somewhat easier since only nuclear families are required. Non-parametric linkage analysis also is more robust because it is unnecessary to specify a model of inheritance for the disease gene. Also, because only affected individuals are sampled (preferably along with their parents), this non-parametric strategy misses the opportunity to extract information from unaffected siblings who could also be recombinant (as shown in Fig. 4.1). Therefore, the LOD score linkage analysis (which is fully parametric) remains the most statistically powerful approach. The robustness of non-parametric linkage analysis, however, has considerable advantages when dealing with complex diseases where there is little justification for assuming any particular model of inheritance despite considerable evidence for some genetic role in the etiology of disease. When dealing with complex diseases, it has been said that showing evidence of linkage is the highest level of statistical evidence that a gene does control risk to disease, because its roots lie in a very specific biological mechanism (Elston, 1981).

For completely informative matings where both parents are heterozygotes for different alleles, estimating IBD sharing between full siblings can be simple (see Fig. 3.3); however, other mating types are less informative and there will be some ambiguity in estimating IBD sharing between siblings. As with LOD score linkage analysis, families vary in their information content, so it becomes important to use highly polymorphic markers to maximize information for linkage analysis. Multi-allelic microsatellites and VNTRs (variable number of tandem repeats) are generally more informative than biallelic single nucleotide polymorphism (SNP) markers, so more parents are likely to be heterozygous and completely informative matings become possible. For this reason, these types of genetic markers were originally preferred for genome-wide linkage analysis. Given advances in genotyping technology, however, dense panels of SNPs are now cheaper. Typically both LOD score and non-parametric linkage are run on subsets of SNPs that are not correlated with one another, because correlated SNPs (i.e. those in strong linkage disequilibrium (LD) with one another) can inflate type I errors in the presence of missing genotypes on family members (Ott *et al.*, 2011).

There are many different statistical tests to assess whether affected sibling pairs share a single marker exactly as expected under the null hypothesis of no linkage (Ziegler and Konig, 2010). Evidence of excess IBD sharing at any one marker corresponds to evidence for linkage to an unobserved gene controlling risk to disease. However, non-parametric linkage analysis does not typically estimate the position of a causal gene; rather it only provides the probability that the null hypothesis of no linkage is correct. Considering multiple markers simultaneously can greatly increase the information content of family data for any form of linkage analysis (LOD score or non-parametric) because more matings will involve "heterozygous" individuals (i.e. those carrying two different haplotypes of alleles across several markers would be a heterozygous diplotype).

## Box 4.1. From LOD Scores to Exome Sequencing

### Breast cancer and the *BRCA1* gene

Perhaps one of the best examples of using LOD score linkage analysis to localize a disease susceptibility gene is the discovery of the *BRCA1* gene for familial breast cancer (Hall *et al.*, 1990). Even before the description of the "common disease/common variant hypothesis" (Risch and Merikangas, 1996), these investigators recognized the challenges for mapping genes controlling complex diseases when they wrote, "Mapping genes for human breast cancer has been complicated by unavoidable epidemiologic realities."

Mapping the *BRCA1* gene was based on a previous segregation analysis (Elston, 1981) using a large, population-based collection of families that gave evidence for a major gene controlling risk of breast cancer with variation in penetrance by age (ranging from 0.37 by age 40 years, 0.66 by age 55 years to 0.82 lifetime risk). The hypothetical risk allele was rare and dominant with a low frequency (0.004–0.02) (Newman *et al.*, 1988).

The authors of the linkage study recruited 23 extended multiplex kindreds, with several members affected with breast cancer, including 146 cases confirmed by pathology reports from surgery, hospital records, and/or death certificates. Genetic relationships among the family members were confirmed using 183 polymorphic markers used in a comprehensive LOD score linkage analysis. This linkage analysis was performed with a VNTR marker on chromosome 17, D17S74, with more than 30 different alleles detected by the size of DNA fragments. This VNTR was highly informative for linkage because its heterozygosity was greater than 90%.

Family 1, the kindred with the strongest evidence of linkage to D17S74 on chromosome 17, is shown in Fig. 4.4a. Among the seven breast cancer cases in this one family, the average age of diagnosis was 33 years. The size alleles of the D17S74 marker are shown as capital letters, and the E allele appears to co-segregate consistently with breast cancer throughout this family. For a $\theta$ of 0.001 (very close linkage), the LOD score for this family alone was 2.36, approaching the conventional statistical threshold of 3.0 for genetic linkage.

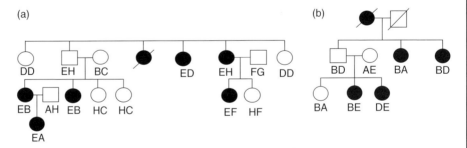

**Fig. 4.4.** (a) Pedigree of Family 1, adapted from Hall *et al.*, 1990. Filled-in symbols are breast cancer cases, and letters are D17S74 alleles by size. The mean age of diagnosis in this family was 33 years, and the LOD score for linkage of breast cancer to D17S74 = 2.36 at $\theta$ = 0.001. (b) Pedigree of Family 2, adapted from Hall *et al.*, 1990. Filled-in symbols are breast cancer cases, and letters are D17S74 alleles by size. Mean age of diagnosis in this family was 37 years, and the LOD score for linkage of breast cancer to D17S74 = 0.50 at $\theta$ = 0.001.

*Continued*

M.A. Austin *et al.*

**Box 4.1.** Continued.

Family 2, with an average age of onset of 37 years and an LOD score of 0.50 at $\theta = 0.001$, is shown in Fig. 4.4b. In this family, there were five cases of breast cancer apparently co-segregating with the B allele at the D17S74 marker, illustrating how different alleles can be linked in different families. In addition, the two affected granddaughters in this family inherited the B allele from their father, who did not develop the disease.

As part of this analysis, LOD scores were computed for each of the remaining 21 kindreds (listed in Table 4.2), with families ranked by the average age of onset in each family. For the first seven such families, with average age of onset ranging from 33 to 45 years, six of the LOD scores were positive, and the cumulative LOD score $(Z(\theta = 0.001))$ was 5.98, providing strong evidence for linkage of early-onset breast cancer to D17S74.

Table 4.2 also shows, however, that there was no evidence of linkage to a gene near D17S74 controlling risk to breast cancer among families with later-onset breast cancer. For families 16 to 23, where ages of onset ranged from 52 to 63, the cumulative LOD score at $\theta = 0.001$ was −5.58, providing strong evidence *against* linkage to this region of chromosome 17. These findings demonstrate *locus heterogeneity* exists for genetic forms of breast cancer, because some families give evidence for linkage to a specific chromosomal region, whereas others do not. Such evidence of locus heterogeneity has been confirmed many times for familial cancer where multiple genes are involved.

The authors (Hall *et al.*, 1990) concluded from these data that "Chromosome 17q21 appears to be the locale of a gene for inherited susceptibility to breast cancer in families with early onset disease." Within 4 years, not only was the *BRCA1* gene identified on the long arm of chromosome 17 (Miki *et al.*, 1994), but a second gene influencing risk to breast cancer (*BRCA2*) was found on chromosome 13 in the same year (Wooster *et al.*, 1994). Taken together, this illustrates how LOD score linkage analysis led to the discovery of two of the most clinically relevant cancer susceptibility genes discovered to date.

**Table 4.2.** LOD scores for linkage of breast cancer to D17S74 by mean age of diagnosis in each family (adapted from Hall *et al.*, 1990).

| Family | Mean age (years) | LOD at $\theta = 0.001$ | Cumulative LOD |
|---|---|---|---|
| 1 | 32.7 | +2.36 | +2.36 |
| 2 | 37.2 | +0.50 | +2.86 |
| 3 | 37.3 | +0.40 | +3.26 |
| 4 | 39.8 | +1.14 | +4.40 |
| 5 | 42.6 | −0.50 | +3.90 |
| 6 | 44.2 | +1.38 | +5.28 |
| 7 | 45.4 | +0.70 | +5.98 |
| 8 to 15 | 47.0 to 51.8 | −1.51 to 0.00 | +2.65 |
| 16 to 23 | 52.0 to 63.3 | −2.71 to +0.65 | −5.48 |

## Exome sequencing in families: the *PALB2* gene

Since these early linkage studies mapping the *BRCA1* and *BRCA2* genes, there has been a growing list of genes associated with moderate increase in risk of breast cancer (Walsh and King, 2007). These include *p53*, *PTEN*, *CHEK2*, *ATM*, *NBSI*, *RAD50*, *BRIP1*, and most recently *PALB2*, the "partner and localizer of *BRCA2*" binding factor

*Continued*

**Box 4.1.** Continued.

that is "crucial for the association of *BRCA2* with chromatin and nuclear structure and for its DNA damage response functions" (Erkko *et al.*, 2007). The *PALB2* gene is located on chromosome 16p12.2 and contains 13 exons, as shown in Fig. 4.5.

At least two studies have shown heterozygosity for a mutation in *PALB2* is associated with increased risk of breast cancer based on sequencing studies. Rahman *et al.* (2007) studied 923 breast cancer cases without recognized *BRCA1* or *BRCA2* mutations. After sequencing the 13 coding exons of the *PALB2* gene, they found five different truncating mutations in the *PALB2* gene among cases and none among 1,084 controls. When taken together, these mutations conferred a 2.3-fold increased risk of being a breast cancer case (P = 0.0025). Erkko *et al.* (2007) studied 113 families from northern Finland who were also negative for *BRCA1*/*BRCA2* mutations, and identified a single founder mutation (c.1592delT) that was consistent with a 2–4-fold increased risk of breast cancer. Similarly, studies of *CHEK2*, *NBS1*, *BRIP1*, *ATM*, and *RAD50* have all demonstrated approximately a 2-fold increased risk associated with breast cancer (Walsh and King, 2007). Walsh and King (2007) note that all of these genes share two important features: (i) a single deleterious mutation in any one of these genes significantly increases breast cancer risk; and (ii) there are many different deleterious mutations in these genes, each of which is individually rare, demonstrating both locus and allelic heterogeneity. They contend these findings are not consistent with a "common disease/common variant" model (Risch and Merikangas, 1996), but rather support a "common disease/multiple rare variant" model.

More recently, Jones and colleagues used exomic sequencing in families to study the role of *PALB2* mutations in familial pancreatic cancer (Jones *et al.*, 2009). They note previous studies have shown tumors from patients with hereditary forms of cancer often have no normal alleles at a causal gene, with one mutation inherited through the germline and the other allele inactivated by a somatic mutation during tumor development. Based on a patient whose tumor DNA had been sequenced, they identified three genes in the patient's germline DNA meeting this criterion, including *PALB2*. They then sought to determine if mutations in *PALB2* were present in 96 additional cases of familial pancreatic cancer from the National Familial Pancreas Tumor Registry (after excluding cases with *BRCA2* mutations). Using DNA from lymphoblastoid cell lines made from blood samples (germline), they sequenced the entire *PALB2* gene.

As shown in Fig. 4.5, these investigators identified three truncating mutations (172–175 del TTGT, 3116 del A, and 3256 C>T) and one intronic variant (IVS5-1 G>T) in the *PALB2* gene among these patients, while no such mutations were reported in a previous analysis of 1,084 normal controls. Among the four families with one person carrying one of these mutations, the 3256 C>T mutation was found in two brothers with early-onset familial pancreatic cancer (Fig. 4.6). The authors conclude "... through complete, unbiased, sequencing of protein coding genes, we have identified a gene responsible for a hereditary disease." Further, they "predict that variation of the approach described here will soon become a standard tool for the discovery of disease-related genes."

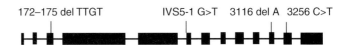

**Fig. 4.5.** Structure of the *PALB2* gene located on chromosome 18q11–18q12. Exons are shown as boxes (not to scale) and germline mutations in familial pancreatic cancer families are shown above (adapted from Jones *et al.*, 2009).

*Continued*

M.A. Austin *et al.*

**Box 4.1.** Continued.

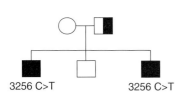

3256 C>T                              3256 C>T

**Fig. 4.6.** Pedigree of a family with familial pancreatic cancer. Filled-in symbols are pancreatic cancer. The two affected brothers, who were both diagnosed in their 50s, have the same truncating mutation in the *PALB2* gene, 3256 C>T. The father had both stomach and prostate cancer (adapted from Jones *et al.*, 2009).

## Summary

Over the last two decades, family studies in genetic epidemiology have evolved from using LOD score linkage analysis to exome sequencing for mapping disease susceptibility genes. These analytical strategies have provided major advances, especially for our understanding of genetic susceptibility to rare, familial forms of common disease.

## 4.2  Family-based Association Studies

### 4.2.1  Linkage and association in families

As described in Section 4.1.1, linkage studies focus on testing hypotheses about the recombination rates ($\theta$) and are always based on families, ranging from large multiplex families spanning three or more generations to pairs of affected siblings drawn from nuclear families. Association studies, however, typically test for differences in allele, genotype, or haplotype frequencies between groups of unrelated people (as in the classic case–control study; see Section 5.4.1) or they test for deviation from Mendelian expectations in transmission of marker alleles within families ascertained through an affected case (as in the transmission disequilibrium test; see Section 4.2.2). In either situation, association tests do not focus on recombination rates (or their consequences) within families, but rather they test a composite null hypothesis of no linkage ($\theta = 0.5$) or no LD, which reflects correlation due to tight linkage between an observed marker allele and an unobserved high-risk allele (see Section 3.5.2).

LD is also termed "gametic phase disequilibrium" and represents a deviation from two-locus Hardy–Weinberg equilibrium (HWE) where allele frequencies at different loci are simple products of the individual allele frequencies. The presence of LD implies allele frequencies at different loci are correlated with one another to some degree. For unlinked loci, admixture between distinct populations can create detectable gametic disequilibrium or deviation from two-locus HWE, but this will fade back toward true equilibrium within ten or fewer generations if there is random mating. If two loci are tightly linked, however, the reduced recombination ($\theta \ll 0.5$) between them allows the LD to persist for many, many generations. Thus, LD is itself a consequence of tight linkage and can be exploited to map genes through association studies using either unrelated individuals or a minimal family structure such as children and their parents.

Ott *et al.* (2011) review the features distinguishing between linkage and association studies, and note the purpose of LOD score-based linkage studies is to estimate recombination fraction directly based on observed or inferred recombinant children from informative matings between parents (which require at least one parent to be a double heterozygote, i.e. heterozygous at the marker and heterozygous at the disease gene). Non-parametric linkage studies also require informative matings, but typically do not estimate the recombination fraction directly, rather relying on the excess sharing of marker alleles by pairs of affected relatives to test the null hypothesis of no linkage. Rejecting this null hypothesis yields evidence of linkage, which can help map causal genes at a relatively course-grained level, i.e. the region of linkage may cover >10 Mb of physical distance. Because association studies rely on LD, which spans much smaller distances (typically in the order of hundreds of kb of physical distance), tests for LD have the advantage of resulting in a much smaller chromosomal region of signal. However, LD is also a complex reflection of the genetic history of the population, and LD blocks do vary across populations. Stable populations that are evolutionarily older will have had more time to approach linkage equilibrium, leading to smaller blocks of LD, making it more difficult to cover the entire genome. In contrast, younger populations will have larger LD blocks spanning greater physical differences, and therefore requiring fewer "tagging" markers to cover the entire genome (see Section 3.5.3).

An intrinsic weakness of linkage analysis is created by the presence of locus heterogeneity (where more than one causal locus exists; see Section 3.2.4). Fortunately, this can be addressed by adding another parameter into the LOD score method described above, although this generates some reduction in statistical power. Similarly, locus heterogeneity will reduce power to map genes using non-parametric linkage methods also, and may broaden the region of signal when (or if) it is detected. Association studies, on the other hand, are susceptible to the detrimental effects of allelic heterogeneity (multiple mutations in the same gene leading to disease) because these multiple mutations are not likely to be in LD with the same markers in and around the gene. Unfortunately, there is currently no analytical strategy to "adjust for" allelic heterogeneity using conventional statistical tests. Therefore, most study designs relying on tests of association reflecting underlying LD must be cautious about interpreting their results from relatively simple statistical tests (see Section 5.3).

### 4.2.2 Case–parent trios and the transmission disequilibrium test (TDT)

Family-based tests of association represent a test of observed versus expected patterns of transmission of marker alleles in families ascertained through a case (or an affected proband). The TDT is one of the original tests and uses the smallest possible family structure: an affected child and his/her parents, also known as a "case–parent trio" or "triad" (Fig. 4.7). In this setting, we are interested in a marker M with two alleles ($M_1$ and $M_2$). This study design uses the TDT for linkage and association between the allele of interest (in this case $M_2$) and disease. This analysis requires that at least one parent in the trio is heterozygous for the marker, denoted as $M_1M_2$.

Under Mendel's law of equal segregation (Section 3.2.1), the $M_1$ and $M_2$ alleles are equally likely to be transmitted from the heterozygote parent to an affected child if the marker is completely independent of any gene controlling risk to disease. If the marker M is linked to and in LD with an unobserved causal gene, we would

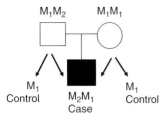

M₁
Control

M₂M₁
Case

M₁
Control

**Fig. 4.7.** Transmission disequilibrium test for a family "trio" with an affected offspring (case) and a heterozygote parent. (Adapted from Speilman *et al.*, 1993.)

expect the $M_2$ allele to be transmitted more often from the heterozygote parent (Fig. 4.7). The underlying hypotheses tested can be written as:

$H_0$: P (Parent transmits $M_2$ | parent is heterozygous $M_1M_2$) = 0.5

$H_1$: P (Parent transmits $M_2$ | parent is heterozygous $M_1M_2$) > 0.5

The TDT simply determines if the segregation of the $M_1$ and $M_2$ alleles is not equal by comparing the frequency of transmitted versus not transmitted alleles. Each case–parent trio contributes two matched case–control pairs to the table, one from each parent, representing a matched pair of transmitted versus non-transmitted alleles (Fig. 4.7). The test compares whether the probability of transmission of the $M_2$ allele from a heterozygous parent to an affected child differs from 0.5. Data for the TDT test can be displayed as shown in Table 4.3, where B is the count of transmitted $M_2$ alleles, C is the count of non-transmitted alleles, and N is the total number of transmitted alleles. Under Mendelian inheritance, these frequencies would be expected to be equal (i.e. B = C in the table).

As described by Spielman *et al.* (1993), the null hypothesis for the allelic TDT test can also be written as:

$H_0$: D (1 − 2θ) = 0

where D = LD and θ = recombination fraction, which represents no LD (i.e. D = 0; see Section 3.5.2) and θ = 0.5 corresponding to no linkage. Thus, D (1 − 2θ) = 0 represents a composite null hypothesis of no linkage or no association between the marker and the hypothesized disease gene (Laird and Lange, 2006). The alternative hypothesis can then be expressed as:

$H_1$: D (1 − 2θ) ≠ 0

That is, there is association (D ≠ 0) *and* linkage (θ ≠ 0.5) between the marker and the disease gene.

Using the layout in Table 4.3, the statistical test for $H_0$ is then a McNemar's test with one degree of freedom:

$\chi^2 = [B - C]^2/[B + C]$

**Table 4.3.** Transmission disequilibrium test for heterozygous ($M_1/M_2$) parents transmitting N alleles (adapted from Spielman *et al.*, 1993).

|  | No. transmitted alleles | | |
| --- | --- | --- | --- |
|  | $M_2$ | $M_1$ | Total |
| Observed | B | C | N |
| Expected | N/2 | N/2 |  |

When this $\chi^2$ test is statistically significant leading to rejection of the composite null hypothesis, we may conclude the $M_2$ allele is transmitted to the affected offspring more or less often than expected under Mendelian inheritance, and thus this marker is linked and associated with some unobserved gene controlling risk to the disease of interest. The TDT test is illustrated in Box 4.2.

---

**Box 4.2. Application: Insulin Gene and Insulin-dependent Diabetes Mellitus (IDDM)**

Spielman *et al.* (1993) presented an allelic TDT test for the class 1 alleles (smallest fragment sizes) at a VNTR marker located within the 5′ region of the insulin gene and risk of type 1 diabetes (IDDM). Among a sample of 94 families with two or more IDDM children, there were 57 heterozygote parents (class 1/other alleles) who transmitted 124 alleles to affected offspring. Of these, 78 alleles (63%) were class 1 and 46 (37%) were other alleles, compared with 62 alleles (50%) each expected under Mendelian inheritance (Table 4.4).

**Table 4.4.** Transmission disequilibrium test for class 1 alleles at a 5′ VNTR marker in the insulin gene and risk of IDDM. (Adapted from Spielman *et al.*, 1993.)

|  | No. transmitted alleles | | |
| --- | --- | --- | --- |
|  | Class 1 | Other | Total |
| Observed | 78 | 46 | 124 |
| Expected | 62 | 62 | |

$$\chi^2 = [78 - 46]^2/[78 + 46] = 8.26, P = 0.004$$

Because this test statistic is significant, these data provide evidence for linkage and association between this marker and a gene controlling risk to IDDM (presumably the insulin gene itself).

---

### 4.2.3 Extensions of the TDT

The original TDT was framed as a comparison between transmitted and non-transmitted alleles and can be viewed as a matched case–control study where transmitted alleles (cases) are simply compared with non-transmitted alleles (controls, Fig. 4.7). It is possible to extend this to genotypes, in which a 3 × 3 table is used to compare genotypes observed in affected children from case–parent trios and check for excess transmission of one or more genotypes. Of course, with larger tables the number of degrees of freedom increases. Schaid (1996) points out such a genotypic TDT can also be framed in a conditional logistic regression model where the observed genotype of the affected child is the case and the three alternative genotypes possible from the parental mating type are "pseudo-controls," leading to a 1:3 matched set for every trio. This approach has some advantages because the unit is now a genotype (corresponding to an individual rather than a chromosome). The conditional logistic regression model allows direct estimation of genotypic relative risks, as well as tests for possible interaction between genotype and some exposure (i.e. gene–environment interaction) or even interaction

M.A. Austin *et al.*

**Box 4.3. Application: Prostate Cancer**

## Introduction and background on prostate cancer genetics

Prostate cancer (PCa) is the leading cause of cancer in US men and the second leading cause of cancer-related deaths (Siegel *et al.*, 2012). Along with age and race, family history is a strong risk factor for the disease. Epidemiological studies demonstrate that men with one or more first-degree affected relatives have a two- to threefold elevation in risk compared with men without any reported family history (Zeegers *et al.*, 2003), and family history profile has been used to stratify three subsets of PCa cases:

**1.** Sporadic: cases with no known family history of the disease, ~75–80% of cases.
**2.** Familial: cases with one first-degree or two second-degree relatives with the disease, ~15–20% of cases.
**3.** Hereditary (HPC): cases with two or more first-degree relatives with the disease, or cases from families in which there are three generations – paternal or maternal lineage – of men with PCa, or cases with at least one first-degree relative with the disease when both were diagnosed with early-onset PCa, ~5% of cases (Carter *et al.*, 1993).

Taken together, observational studies, twin studies, segregation studies, and family-based linkage studies provide strong evidence of an inherited component to the etiology of PCa, with 42% of disease incidence estimated to be due to genetic predisposition (Lichtenstein *et al.*, 2000). Recent studies have begun to elucidate some of the genetic variants and mutations that contribute to PCa susceptibility.

Over the past decade, research efforts to discover common, low-penetrant genetic variants as well as rare, moderate- to high-penetrant genetic mutations that play a role in PCa risk have intensified. Genome-wide association studies (GWAS; see Chapter 5) of common variants (minor allele frequency, MAF > 5–10%) have identified more than 70 risk-associated loci (each with a modest relative risk, RR ~1.2) for PCa. Combined, these genetic risk factors are estimated to account for ~30% of the genetic component of the disease (Varghese and Easton, 2010; Eeles *et al.*, 2013). Published GWAS focused on sporadic PCa cases, but familial cases were also represented. Family-based linkage studies have also identified more than two dozen putative loci for HPC with "significant" or "suggestive" signals from linkage analysis. Many of these loci, however, have not been confirmed in independent studies and have not yielded evidence of specific mutations (Easton *et al.*, 2003; Ostrander *et al.*, 2004). Several challenges to finding HPC genes are probably responsible, including disease heterogeneity, locus heterogeneity, and incomplete penetrance. Recent technological advances such as denser genome-wide arrays and next-generation sequencing, as well as more refined study designs, are beginning to yield novel insights into PCa susceptibility.

## The PROGRESS study

The *Prostate Cancer Genetic Research Study* (PROGRESS) was initiated in 1995 with the goal of recruiting families with a defined pattern of HPC for linkage studies aimed at mapping genes for HPC. Families were ascertained from across North America through public media (television, radio, newspaper, and magazine advertisements) and contact with members of relevant professional organizations (e.g. the American Urology Association, other PCa support groups).

*Continued*

---

**Box 4.3.** Continued.

Most families were self-referred and were initially enrolled through an index family member who called the study's publicized toll-free number, and who was asked to provide details regarding the family's history of PCa (e.g. number of affected individuals, ages at diagnosis, relationship among affected individuals, and their vital status). These data were reviewed by a team of researchers who determined eligibility under the HPC criteria described above. The representative or index member of each eligible family was mailed a letter describing the study, a study brochure, and a form ascertaining contact information and permission to contact relevant male and female family members. Through this approach, all affected men, unaffected men aged 40 years and older, and selected women were invited to enroll in the study. All eligible individuals within each family were asked to complete a baseline questionnaire covering details of their medical history and family cancer history and to provide a blood sample for genetic studies. Two follow-up surveys have been completed at about 5 and 10 years after initial study enrollment to update medical and cancer history information. In addition, a *PROGRESS Newsletter* is sent to all participants once a year to provide feedback on completed and ongoing study activities and updates on prostate cancer genetic research findings, as well as a reminder to contact the study regarding any new cancer diagnoses within the family.

To date, a total of 307 HPC families have joined PROGRESS, with an average of 7.6 members per family participating. There are currently 1,085 affected men (living and deceased), 675 unaffected men, and 588 women in the study. The majority of these families are of European descent (n = 289).

## Linkage analysis: the challenges of disease and locus heterogeneity

Two genome-wide linkage studies have been completed on PROGRESS families, the first based on genotyping of 441 microsatellite markers and the second based on genotyping of ~6,000 SNP markers (Janer *et al.*, 2003; Stanford *et al.*, 2009). The latter effort identified overall suggestive evidence for linkage at 7q21 (heterogeneity LOD, HLOD = 1.87 (Ott, 1999)), 8q22 (non-parametric Kong and Cox LOD, KCLOD = 1.88 (Kong and Cox, 1997)) and 15q13–q14 (HLOD = 1.99) in families of European ancestry, and nominal evidence of linkage at 2q24 (LOD = 1.73) in the 12 African–American HPC families. In an effort to address disease heterogeneity, clinical features of aggressive PCa were utilized to create a more homogeneous subset of families in which at least two men were diagnosed with high Gleason score tumors, advanced stage, diagnostic prostate-specific antigen (PSA) >20 ng/ml, or who died of PCa before age 65. Analysis of the 126 families with multiple men with an aggressive PCa phenotype highlighted additional linkage regions, and when early age at diagnosis (age <65 years) was also considered, the linkage signal on 15q13–q14 (KCLOD = 2.82) became more suggestive for a locus harboring an HPC gene mutation (Stanford *et al.*, 2009).

Another approach to reduce locus heterogeneity when dealing with a complex disease such as PCa is to consider the presence of other primary cancers in the family. This strategy has been used successfully to stratify PROGRESS families for linkage analyses into subsets with HPC and primary brain cancer (Gibbs *et al.*, 1999), kidney cancer (Johanneson *et al.*, 2007), pancreas cancer (Pierce *et al.*, 2007), or colon cancer (FitzGerald *et al.*, 2010). In the latter analysis of HPC–colon cancer families, the

*Continued*

M.A. Austin *et al.*

**Box 4.3.** Continued.

strongest linkage signal was identified at 15q14 when individuals with both PCa and colon cancer were coded as affected in the subset of 27 HPC families with at least two members with colon cancer (recessive HLOD = 3.88).

These results and other published data illustrate how strategies such as using clinical data (e.g. to define early-onset or more aggressive PCa phenotypes) and family characteristics (e.g. presence of other primary cancers) may create more homogeneous subsets of HPC families and can be helpful for identification of genetic linkage, which is otherwise challenging due to both disease and locus heterogeneity. Another strategy is to pool data across multiple studies to enhance statistical power for finding linkage in defined subsets of families (e.g. those with multiple PCa cases with an aggressive phenotype, or those with five or more affected men).

## International Consortium for Prostate Cancer Genetics (ICPCG)

In 1998, a number of groups with collections of HPC families from North America, Australia, Finland, Norway, Sweden, and the UK came together to form the ICPCG. The first ICPCG combined analyses included 772 HPC families and evaluated a putative linkage region on 1q24–25, for which the data failed to provide confirmatory evidence (Xu *et al.*, 2000). As shown in Table 4.5, the next ICPCG effort included 1,233 HPC families, and revealed significant linkage at 22q12 (LOD = 3.57) in HPC families with at least five affected members (Xu *et al.*, 2005). Interestingly, the locus at 22q12 was also highlighted in two other linkage studies when the analyses considered only men with an aggressive PCa phenotype (based on Gleason score, stage, diagnostic PSA, and early death from PCa) (Chang *et al.*, 2005; Stanford *et al.*, 2006). Follow-up fine-mapping studies of this 22q12 locus narrowed the region to a 15 kb interval spanning only one gene, *Apolipoprotein L3* (*APOL3*); and SNPs in the 3′ end of this gene were significantly associated with PCa in two HPC family datasets and in an independent population-based case–control dataset (Johanneson *et al.*, 2010).

**Table 4.5.** Chromosomal locations and LOD scores for linkage analysis from the ICPCG based on 1,233 families with hereditary prostate cancer (adapted from Xu *et al.*, 2005).

| Locus (LOD score) | | |
| --- | --- | --- |
| Main analysis | ≥5 Affected | ≤ Age 65 at diagnosis |
| 5q12 (2.28) | 1q25 (2.62) | 3p24 (2.37) |
| 8p21 (1.97) | 8q13 (2.41) | 5q35 (2.05) |
| 15q11 (2.10) | 13q14 (2.27) | 11q22 (2.20) |
| 17q21 (1.99) | 16q13 (1.88) | Xq12 (2.30) |
| 22q12 (1.95) | 17q21 (2.04) | |
| | 22q12 (3.57) | |

*Continued*

**Box 4.3.** Continued.

## Next-generation sequencing projects

With advances in sequencing technology (see Section 3.6), efforts have shifted toward sequencing of targeted regions and whole-exome sequencing (WES), with the goal of identifying rare causal mutations. To optimize the chance of finding such susceptibility genes and their underlying mutations, especially those with rare allele frequencies, Cirulli and Goldstein (2010) propose three study design strategies: (i) using whole-genome or whole-exome sequencing; (ii) sequencing multiple cases within a family; and/or (iii) sequencing cases with an extreme phenotype (e.g. more aggressive features of disease, early onset). Another issue to consider in the design of WES projects is who to select for sequencing. There are ~3 million single nucleotide variants (SNVs) in an individual's genome and of these ~80–90% will be common variants found in HapMap or the 1000 Genomes Project (see Chapter 9). After filtering WES data against these public SNP databases, one can expect to identify ~300 private non-synonymous variants in an individual of European descent. Sequencing two affected first cousins, who will share ~1/8 of their genome IBD, can reduce the number of private variants they are likely to share to 300/8 = ~38; this is further reduced to 300/64 = ~5 if three first cousins are sequenced. This strategy is expected to reduce the number of candidate mutations that will require follow-up in validation studies. These guidelines have been helpful in designing next-generation sequencing studies of HPC, which are beginning to find novel susceptibility genes.

The recent discovery of a mutation (G84E) in the *HOXB13* gene is an example of how using next-generation sequencing technology can lead to discovery of rare mutations in previously defined linkage regions (Ewing *et al.*, 2012). To follow up on a linkage peak on 17q21–22, germline DNA from 94 unrelated PCa cases representing 94 HPC families was used to sequence across 200 genes within the region. A variant in *HOXB13* was found to co-segregate with PCa in four of the 94 families, and was more common in cases with early-onset, familial PCa (3.1%) compared with cases with later-onset, non-familial PCa (0.6%), and was rare (0.1%) in men without any family history of PCa. These results have been confirmed by the larger ICPCG collaborative group (Xu *et al.*, 2013). A similar effort is currently underway within PROGRESS families and other selected ICPCG families involving targeted sequencing across the linkage region on 15q13.3–q14. As described above, an initial linkage peak was observed in analyses of early-onset, more aggressive PCa in HPC families, as well as the subset of PROGRESS families with both HPC and colon cancer.

To identify the underlying 15q13.3–q14 HPC susceptibility gene, a study utilizing next-generation sequencing technology was undertaken. The study involves resequencing multiple members from nine PROGRESS and five ICPCG families with evidence of linkage to 15q13.3–q14. For this effort, two to three distantly related affected men with a shared "disease haplotype" were selected for sequencing. This approach is expected to increase the probability of observing an actual disease-associated mutation rather than a variant shared IBD, and reduce the number of candidate mutations that will require follow-up. In addition, one relative without a shared "disease haplotype" was selected for sequencing to reduce the number of candidate mutations for follow-up by filtering family-specific variants and reduce the number of false positives arising through sequencing artifacts. Sequencing has been completed and the analyses are currently underway. Results of this effort as well as other targeted sequencing endeavors are expected soon.

*Continued*

M.A. Austin *et al.*

**Box 4.3.** Continued.

WES projects have also been initiated by several of the ICPCG groups to identify rare mutations for HPC (Cirulli and Goldstein, 2010). One such effort within PROGRESS has focused on sequencing individuals (80 affected, 11 unaffected) from 19 Caucasian HPC families with five or more affected men in which there are multiple cases diagnosed with an aggressive phenotype and/or early-onset PCa. After filtering these data, 196 candidate mutations, including 174 SNVs and 22 indels, were prioritized for follow-up. SNVs were filtered on a family-level basis using four different methods, some of which allowed for incomplete penetrance and phenocopies, as well as two MAF criteria (i.e. <0.01 and <0.02). Filtered SNVs were further prioritized according to type (nonsense < splice site < missense), prediction scores for likely deleterious effects, and presence within a previously identified linkage region for HPC. Indels were also filtered on a family-level basis, and the four data filters allowed for no, one, two, and three phenocopies. Indels were removed from further consideration if they were observed in any unaffected men. Filtered indels were then further prioritized by type (frameshift < UTR < non-frameshift), location, and presence within a prior linkage region. Molecular inversion probe assays were successfully designed for 130 of the candidate mutations, and have been used to genotype all affected and unaffected men with DNA available in an independent set of 270 Caucasian HPC families for validation. Analyses are underway and results are expected soon (FitzGerald *et al.*, unpublished results).

**Summary**

Advances in sequencing technology and study design are beginning to yield important new insights into the genetics of HPC, and some HPC-associated mutations are also turning out to be risk alleles for sporadic PCa (e.g. the G84E mutation in the *HOXB13* gene). Over the next several years, these advances are expected to substantially expand our knowledge and concept of the genetic susceptibility to PCa. The hope is that these molecular discoveries will ultimately lead to better ways to diagnose, treat, and prevent this common and complex disease.

between genotypes at separate loci (i.e. gene–gene interaction). Schwender *et al.* (2012) recently developed a closed form solution to this conditional logistic regression by taking advantage of the limited number of Mendelian possibilities, thereby bypassing the need for iterative likelihood-based model fitting to improve the computational time. Weinberg *et al.* (1998) also developed a likelihood-based approach for a genotypic TDT for both child and mother simultaneously in the context of log-linear models where genotypic relative risks associated with an individual marker or haplotypes of several markers can be estimated (Gjessing and Lie, 2006).

Laird and Lange (2006) review a generalized family-based association test (FBAT), which offers a test for independence between genetic markers and observed phenotypes and provides a flexible approach to consider both case–parent trios and nuclear family data. This FBAT is identical to the genotypic TDT when the sample consists only of independent case–parent trios, but can also incorporate multiple children (i.e. siblings of the cases) into the analysis. Although this FBAT approach requires specifying a model of inheritance for the phenotype, it does offer a systematic test for the composite null hypothesis of no linkage and no LD, and rejecting this null hypothesis implies markers (individual SNPs or haplotypes of several SNPs) in a specific region of the genome are linked and in LD with an unobserved causal gene.

A variety of other extensions to the TDT have been developed, including methods for continuous phenotypes (Allison, 1997; Rabinowitz, 1997), an approach for use in sibships with at least one affected and one unaffected individual (Spielman and Ewens, 1998), a test for when only one parent is available (Sun *et al.*, 1999), tests for X-linked inheritance where only mothers can be informative, and a test in general pedigrees (Martin *et al.*, 2000). An up-to-date summary of the available tests is provided by Ott *et al.* (2011).

## 4.3   Conclusion

Family studies remain a fundamental component of genetic epidemiology for finding disease susceptibility genes. LOD score linkage analysis counts recombinant and non-recombinant offspring to search for evidence of co-segregation between a hypothetical disease gene and a known genetic marker. Because informative, multi-generational families can be difficult to ascertain, non-parametric linkage analysis, based on excess sharing of marker alleles IBD between relatives, especially siblings, can be a useful alternative analysis approach. Genetic association studies can also be conducted in families, often using parent–offspring trios, by testing for deviations from Mendelian expectations in the transmission of marker alleles using the TDT test.

Over the past two decades, family studies in genetic epidemiology have evolved from using linkage analysis to exome and whole-genome sequencing for finding disease susceptibility genes. These analytical strategies have provided major advances for our understanding of genetic susceptibility to rare, familial forms of common disease, as well as common, complex diseases such as prostate cancer. The goal of all of the approaches is to use molecular discoveries to better diagnose, treat, and prevent disease.

## Acknowledgments

The PROGRESS study is supported by the National Cancer Institute, NIH (R01 CA080122), with additional support from the Fred Hutchinson Cancer Research Center and the Prostate Cancer Foundation.

## Further Reading

Cirulli, E.T. and Goldstein, D.B. (2010) Uncovering the roles of rare variants in common disease through whole-genome sequencing. *Nature Reviews Genetics* 11, 415–425.

Khoury, M.J., Beaty, T.H. and Cohen, B.H. (1993) *Fundamentals of Genetic Epidemiology*. Oxford University Press, New York.

Ott, J. (1999) *Analysis of Human Genetic Linkage*, 3rd edn. The Johns Hopkins University Press, Baltimore and London.

M.A. Austin *et al.*

Wang, S.S., Beaty, T.H. and Khoury, M.J. (2010) Genetic epidemiology. In: Speicher, M.R., Antonarakis, S.E., Motulsky, A.G., Vogel, F. and Motulsky, A.G. (eds) *Vogel and Motulsky's Human Genetics. Problems and Approaches*, 4th edn. Springer-Verlag, Berlin, pp. 617–634.

# References

Allison, D.B. (1997) Transmission disequilibrium tests for quantitative traits. *American Journal of Human Genetics* 60, 676–690.

Carter, B.S., Bova, G.S., Beaty, T.H., Steinberg, G.D., Childs, B., Isaacs, W.B. and Walsh, P.C. (1993) Hereditary prostate cancer: epidemiologic and clinical features. *Journal of Urology* 150, 797–802.

Chang, B.L., Isaacs, S.D., Wiley, K.E., Gillanders, E.M. and Zheng, S.L. (2005) Genome-wide screen for prostate cancer susceptibility genes in men with clinically significant disease. *Prostate* 64, 356–361.

Cirulli, E.T. and Goldstein, D.B. (2010) Uncovering the roles of rare variants in common disease through whole-genome sequencing. *Nature Reviews Genetics* 11, 415–425.

Easton, D.F., Schaid, D.J., Whittemore, A.S., Isaacs, W.J. and International Consortium for Prostate Cancer Genetics (2003) Where are the prostate cancer genes? A summary of eight genome wide searches. *Prostate* 57, 261–269.

Eeles, R.A., Olama, A.A., Benlloch, S., Saunders, E.J., Leongamornlert, D.A., Tymrakiewicz, M. *et al.* (2013) Identification of 23 new prostate cancer susceptibility loci using the iCOGS custom genotyping array. *Nature Genetics* 45, 385–391.

Elston, R.C. (1981) Segregation analysis. *Advances in Human Genetics* 11, 63–120

Erkko, H., Xia, B., Nikklia, J., Schleutker, J., Syrjakoski, K., Mannermaa, A., *et al.* (2007) A recurrent mutation in PALB2 in Finnish cancer families. *Nature* 466, 316–319.

Ewing, C.M., Ray, A.M., Lange, E.M., Zuhlke, K.A., Robbins, C.M., Tembe, W.D., *et al.* (2012) Germline mutations in *HOXB13* and prostate-cancer risk. *New England Journal of Medicine* 366, 141–149.

FitzGerald, L.M., McDonnell, S.K., Carlson, E.E., Langeberg, W., McIntosh, L.M., Deutsch K., *et al.* (2010) Genome-wide linkage analyses of hereditary prostate cancer families with colon cancer provide further evidence for a prostate cancer susceptibility locus on 15q11–q14. *European Journal of Human Genetics* 18, 1141–1147.

Gibbs, M., Stanford, J.L., McIndoe, R.A., Jarvik, G.P., Kolb, S., Goode, E.L., *et al.* (1999) Evidence for a rare prostate cancer-susceptibility locus at chromosome 1p36. *American Journal of Human Genetics* 64, 776–787.

Gjessing, H.K. and Lie R.T. (2006) Case–parent triads: estimating single- and double-dose effects of fetal and maternal disease gene haplotypes. *Annals of Human Genetics* 70, 382–396.

Hall, J.M., Lee, M.K., Newman, B., Morrow, J.E., Anderson, L.A., Huey, B. and King, M.-C. (1990) Linkage of early-onset familial breast cancer to chromosome 17q21. *Science* 250, 1684–1689.

Janer, M., Friedrichsen, D.M., Stanford, J.L., Badzioch, M.D., Kolb, S., Deutsch, K., *et al.* (2003) Genomic scan of 254 hereditary prostate cancer families. *Prostate* 57, 309–319.

Johanneson, B., Deutsch, K., McIntosh, L., Friedrichsen-Karyadi, D.M., Janer, M., Kwon, E.M., *et al.* (2007) Suggestive genetic linkage to chromosome 11p11.2–q12.2 in hereditary prostate cancer families with primary kidney cancer. *Prostate* 67, 732–742.

Johanneson, B., McDonnell, S.K., Karyadi, D.M., Quignon, P., McIntosh, L., *et al.* (2010) Family-based association analysis of 42 hereditary prostate cancer families identifies the *Apolipoprotein L3* region on chromosome 22q12 as a risk locus. *Human Molecular Genetics* 19, 3852–3862.

Jones, S., Hruban, R.H., Kamiyama, M., Borges, M., Zhang, X., Parsons, D.W., *et al.* (2009) Exomic sequencing identifies *PALB2* as a pancreatic cancer susceptibility gene. *Science* 324, 217.

Khoury, M.J., Beaty, T.H., Cohen, B.H., with Meyers D.A. (1993) Epidemiologic approaches to familial aggregation III. Linkage analysis. In: Khoury, M.J., Beaty, T.H. and Cohen, B.H. (eds) *Fundamentals of Genetic Epidemiology*. Oxford University Press, New York, pp. 284–311.

Kong, A. and Cox, N.J. (1997) Allele-sharing methods: LOD scores and accurate linkage tests. *American Journal of Human Genetics* 61, 1179–1188.

Laird, N.M. and Lange, C. (2006) Family-based designs in the age of large-scale gene-association studies. *Nature Reviews Genetics* 7, 385–394.

Lichtenstein, P., Holm, N.V., Verkasalo, P.K., Iliadou, A., Kaprio, J., Koskenvuo, M., *et al.* (2000) Environmental and heritable factors in the causation of cancer – analyses of cohorts of twins from Sweden, Denmark, and Finland. *New England Journal of Medicine* 343, 78–85.

Martin, E.R., Monks, S.A., Warren, L.L. and Kaplan, N.L. (2000) A test for linkage and association in general pedigrees: the pedigree disequilibrium test. *American Journal of Human Genetics* 67, 146–154.

Miki, Y., Swensen, J., Shattuck-Eidens, D., Futreal, P.A., Harshman, K., Tavtigian, S., *et al.* (1994) A strong candidate for the breast and ovarian cancer susceptibility gene *BRCA1*. *Science* 266, 66–71.

Newman, B., Austin, M.A., Lee, M. and King, M.-C. (1988) Inheritance of human breast cancer: evidence for autosomal dominant transmission in high-risk families. *Proceedings of the National Academy of Sciences USA* 85, 3044–3048.

Ostrander, E.A., Markianos, K. and Stanford, J.L. (2004) Finding prostate cancer susceptibility genes. *Annual Review of Genomics and Human Genetics* 5, 151–175.

Ott, J. (1999) *Analysis of Human Genetic Linkage*, 3rd edn. The Johns Hopkins University Press, Baltimore and London, pp. 114–150.

Ott, J., Kamatani, Y. and Lathrop, M. (2011) Family-based designs for genome-wide association studies. *Nature Reviews Genetics* 12, 465–474.

Pierce, B.L., Friedrichsen-Karyadi, D.M., McIntosh, L., Deutsh, K., Hood, L., Ostrander, E.A., *et al.* (2007) Genomic scan of 12 hereditary prostate cancer families having an occurrence of pancreas cancer. *Prostate* 67, 410–415.

Rabinowitz, D. (1997) A transmission disequilibrium test for quantitative trait loci. *Human Heredity* 47, 342–350.

Rahman, N., Seal, S., Thompson, D., Kelly, P., Renwick, A., Elliott, A., *et al.* (2007) *PALB2*, which encodes a *BRCA2*-interaction protein, is a breast cancer susceptibility gene. *Nature Genetics* 39, 165–167.

Risch, N. and Merikangas, K. (1996) The future of genetic studies of complex human diseases. *Science* 273, 1516–1517.

Schaid, D.J. (1996) General score tests for associations of genetic markers with disease using cases and their parents. *Genetic Epidemiology* 13, 423–449.

Schwender, H., Taub, M.A., Beaty, T.H., Marazita, M.L. and Ruczinski, I. (2012) Rapid testing of SNPs and gene–environment interactions in case–parent trio data based on exact analytical parameter estimation. *Biometrics* 68, 766–773.

Siegel, R., Naishadham, D. and Jemal, A (2012) Cancer statistics, 2012. *CA: A Cancer Journal for Clinicians* 62, 10–29.

Spielman, R.S. and Ewens, W.J. (1998) A sibship test for linkage in the presence of association: the sib transmission/disequilibrium test. *American Journal of Human Genetics* 62, 450–458.

Spielman, R.S., McGinnis, R.E. and Ewens, W.J. (1993) Transmission test for linkage disequilibrium: the insulin gene region and insulin-dependent diabetes mellitus (IDDM). *American Journal of Human Genetics* 52, 506–516.

Stanford, J.L., McDonnell, S.K., Friedrichsen, D.M., Carlson, E.E., Kolb, S., Deutsch, K., *et al.* (2006) Prostate cancer and genetic susceptibility: a genome scan incorporating disease aggressiveness. *Prostate* 66, 317–325.

Stanford, J.L., FitzGerald, L.M., McDonnell, S.K., Carlson, E.E., McIntosh, L.M., Deutsch, K., *et al.* (2009) Dense genome-wide SNP linkage scan in 301 hereditary prostate cancer families identifies multiple regions with suggestive evidence for linkage. *Human Molecular Genetics* 18, 1839–1848

Sun, F., Flanders, W.D., Yang, Q. and Khoury, M.J. (1999) Transmission disequilibrium test (TDT) when only one parent is available: the 1-TDT. *American Journal of Epidemiology* 150, 97–104.

Varghese, J.S. and Easton, D.F. (2010) Genome-wide association studies in common cancers – what have we learnt? *Current Opinion in Genetics & Development* 20, 201–209.

Walsh, T. and King, M.-C. (2007) Ten genes for inherited breast cancer. *Cancer Cell* 11, 103–105.

Weinberg, C.R., Wilcox, A.J. and Lie, R.T. (1998) A log-linear approach to case–parent-triad data: assessing effects of disease genes that act either directly or through maternal effects and that may be subject to parental imprinting. *American Journal of Human Genetics* 62, 969–978.

Wooster, R., Neuhausen, S.L., Mangion, J., Quirk, Y., Ford, D., Collins, N., *et al.* (1994) Localization of a breast cancer susceptibility gene, BRCA2, to chromosome 13q12-13. *Science* 265, 2088–2090.

Xu, J. (2000) Combined analysis of hereditary prostate cancer linkage to *1q24-25*: results from 772 hereditary prostate cancer families from the International Consortium for Prostate Cancer Genetics. *American Journal of Human Genetics* 66, 945–957.

Xu, J., Dimitrov, L., Chang, B.L., Adams, T.S., Turner, A.R., Meyers, D.A., *et al.* (2005) A combined genomewide linkage scan of 1,233 families for prostate cancer-susceptibility genes conducted by the International Consortium for Prostate Cancer Genetics. *American Journal of Human Genetics* 77, 219–229.

Xu, J., Lange, E.M., Lu, L., Zheng, S.L., Wang, Z., Thibodeau, S.N. *et al.* (2013) *HOXB13* is a susceptibility gene for prostate cancer: results from the International Consortium for Prostate Cancer Genetics. *Human Genetics* 132, 5–14.

Zeegers, M.P.A., Jellema, A. and Ostrer, H. (2003) Empiric risk of prostate carcinoma for relatives of patients with prostate carcinoma: a meta-analysis. *Cancer* 97, 1894–1903.

Ziegler, A. and Konig, I.R. (2010) Model-free linkage analysis. In: *A Statistical Approach to Genetic Epidemiology. Concepts and Applications*, 2nd edn. Wylie-VCH Verlag GmbH & Co. KGaA, Weinheim, pp. 189–220.

# 5 Genetic Association Studies

MELISSA A. AUSTIN, M.S., PH.D.,[1]
BRUCE M. PSATY, M.D., PH.D.,[2]
AND STEPHEN M. SCHWARTZ, PH.D., M.P.H.[3]

[1]*Department of Epidemiology, University of Washington, Seattle, Washington;* [2]*Cardiovascular Health Research Unit, Departments of Medicine, Epidemiology, and Health Services, University of Washington and Group Health Research Institute, Group Health Cooperative, Seattle, Washington;* [3]*Division of Public Health Sciences, Fred Hutchinson Cancer Research Center, and Department of Epidemiology, University of Washington, Seattle, Washington*

## Synopsis

- Based on the "common disease/common variant" hypothesis, genetic epidemiologists undertake genetic association studies to search for susceptibility genes for complex diseases, using either candidate gene or genome-wide approaches. Both approaches can use case–control, cohort, and case–parent trio designs, and can employ a variety of genetic markers.

- In the candidate gene approach, genes whose functions are known or suspected to be involved in disease predisposition, and specific polymorphisms within those genes, are studied.

- Genome-wide association studies (GWAS) examine genetic markers that span the entire genome in order to identify new genes or confirm previously known susceptibility genes. They use high-throughput technologies for genotyping millions of single nucleotide polymorphisms (SNPs). In order to have sufficient statistical power to detect the small effect sizes found in most GWAS, very large samples are used, often based on large-scale collaborations.

- Interpretation of genetic association results is complex and can be attributable to: a direct, causal relationship; an indirect relationship due to linkage disequilibrium; false-positive associations due to multiple comparisons, departure from Hardy–Weinberg equilibrium, and/or population stratification; false negatives due to inadequate statistical power, small effect sizes, and /or insufficient genomic coverage.

- The Cohorts for Heart and Aging Research in Genomic Epidemiology (CHARGE) Consortium is an example of an effective and productive GWAS collaboration that takes advantage of the hundreds of millions of dollars invested in National Institute of Health (NIH)-funded cohort studies. It represents an innovative model of investigator-initiated collaborative research to identify genetic loci associated with a variety of cardiovascular and aging phenotypes.

- Although more than 2,000 SNPs have been associated with complex traits and diseases to date based on GWAS, these associations do not explain most of the heritability of these traits. Using height as an example, possible reasons for this "missing heritability" are considered.

© M.A. Austin 2013. *Genetic Epidemiology: Methods and Applications*
(M.A. Austin *et al.*)

- Advances in DNA sequencing, especially exome sequencing, are being used to detect associations between rare genetic variants and common diseases based on new study designs and statistical analysis approaches that allow more direct identification of causal variants.

## 5.1 Introduction to Genetic Association Studies

The recognition that genetic association studies can be statistically more powerful than family-based linkage analysis in identifying genes for common, complex diseases led to the "common disease/common variant" (CDCV) hypothesis in the 1990s (Risch and Merikangas, 1996). Since then, this hypothesis has been the basis for both candidate gene and genome-wide association studies (GWAS) (Visscher *et al.*, 2012). In addition, certain disease gene relationships can only be studied using association (such as studies of the mitochrondrial genome; see Chapter 8), conducting family studies may not be feasible in many settings, and genetic association studies can make use of well-developed traditional epidemiologic study designs.

The candidate gene approach and the genome-wide approach are complementary strategies for testing the CDCV hypothesis through genetic association studies. In the candidate gene approach, the etiologic mechanism(s) may be known or suspected, the physiologic effectors of the mechanism(s) may be known, and variation in genes whose functions are players in the mechanisms are studied. In contrast, the genome-wide approach is often referred to as "agnostic" because it ignores known etiologic mechanisms and physiology and examines genetic markers that span the entire genome. These types of studies can identify disease susceptibility genes that had not been contemplated as having a role in the disease, and may also confirm previously identified candidate genes.

Both approaches can use case–control, cohort, and case–parent trio designs, and can employ a variety of genetic markers, including single nucleotide polymorphisms (SNPs), microsatellites, and/or copy number variants. However, unlike genetic linkage studies that seek to identify the location of a susceptibility gene on a chromosome based on families, all genetic association studies evaluate the relationship between a specific allele and risk of disease and, with the exception of the case–parent trio design, are based on genetically unrelated study participants.

More recently, the alternative "common disease/rare variant" (CDRV) hypothesis has been described (Li and Leal, 2008). Rather than complex diseases being explained by common genomic variants with small effect sizes, this theory proposes that genetic control of common diseases is due to multiple rare, deleterious variants with strong impact (Cirulli and Goldstein, 2010). DNA sequence data, including exome sequencing results, can be used to address this hypothesis, and new study designs and statistical methods are being developed to assess these associations.

## 5.2 Study Designs for Candidate Gene Studies

### 5.2.1 Practical considerations for selecting candidate genes

The first step in conducting a candidate gene study is to identify genes that may be involved in the disease or phenotype of interest. As Tabor *et al.* (2002) have described, the process usually begins by examining the published studies of the phenotype for suggestions of genes that have been previously related to the phenotype, and determining whether there are functional variants of these genes. This literature may include animal models and/or expression studies in tissues or cells, not only human studies. Other possibilities include genes and proteins that process pathogens, carcinogens, or environmental risk factors relevant to the etiology of the disease.

Next, polymorphisms in the selected genes must be chosen. The traditional definition of a genetic polymorphism is a variant with a minor allele frequency of at least 1% in the population (Gelehrter et al., 1998; Costa and Eaton, 2006). This term is, however, generally used to refer to variation in the genome, especially with the recent emphasis on the importance of "rare" variants in relation to disease risk (Cirulli and Goldstein, 2010). Because SNPs occur approximately every 500 to 1,000 bp in the genome, and are relatively easy to genotype, these are the most often used type of polymorphisms in association studies. However, structural variations, including copy number variants, insertions and deletions ("indels"), chromosomal inversions, and translocations, as well as VNTRs (variable number of tandem repeats), can be used. Even with recent advances in genomic technology, it may be necessary to prioritize SNPs for genotyping in candidate gene studies. For SNPs that are located in coding regions, Tabor et al. (2002) recommend the following priorities for selecting types of variant polymorphisms:

1. Nonsense (results in premature termination of an amino acid sequence by insertion of a stop codon).
2. Missense/non-synonymous, non-conservative (changes an amino acid in a protein to one with different biochemical properties).
3. Missense/non-synonymous, conservative (changes an amino acid in a protein to one with similar properties).
4. Insertions/deletions ("indels") or frameshift (may result in codon change and thus disrupt the amino acid sequence).
5. Sense/synonymous or "silent" mutations (do not change amino acids in the protein due to redundancy of the genetic code, but can cause changes in conformation, expression, and function of proteins (Sauna and Kimchi-Sarfaty, 2011))

Other types of variants can occur outside the coding region, including:

6. Promoter/regulatory regions: promoter, 5′ UTR, or 3′ UTR.
7. Splice sites/intron–exon boundaries.
8. Intronic: regions within introns.
9. Intergenic: regions between genes.

Although variants in these regions do not code for proteins, they can be useful as tag SNPs to identify regions of the genome, or variants within candidate genes, that may be in linkage disequilibrium (LD) with a causal disease variant (see Section 3.5). In fact, most of the SNPs found to be associated with disease in GWAS to date are in these types of non-coding regions (Manolio, 2010). Rapid advances in genome sciences are demonstrating that, in addition to serving as tags, these regions in themselves are important functional elements in the human genome (Lander, 2012), demonstrated by recent publications from the Encyclopedia of DNA Elements (ENCODE) consortium (Nature ENCODE Explorer, 2012).

Box 5.1 provides examples of a candidate gene association study that investigated the relationships between genes encoding coagulation factors and risk of cardiovascular disease.

M.A. Austin *et al.*

## Box 5.1. Application: Coagulation Factors and Cardiovascular Disease

In humans, the balance between blood coagulation and anti-coagulation is delicately maintained through pathways featuring cascades of enzymes, deficiencies of which (such as Factor VIII and Factor IX) have long been known to be caused by rare mutations and lead to hemophilia. In contrast, genetic variation that promotes clotting, and thus would be a risk factor for diseases in which clotting is a key mechanism (e.g. venous thrombosis and myocardial infarction), have only more recently been identified. Factor V normally becomes activated when clotting is needed, because activated Factor V in combination with activated Factor X promotes the formation of fibrin (polymers of which form the basis of clots) via activation of thrombin from prothrombin (Factor II). Factor V is maintained in an inactive (anti-coagulogenic) state through cleavage by activated Protein C (APC). In the mid-1990s, researchers using classic genetic epidemiology methods coupled with biochemical and molecular genetic investigations identified SNPs in both Factor V and Factor II that alter the function of these enzymes to tip the balance towards a pro-coagulation phenotype. Factor V Arg506Gln (rs6025), with a minor allele frequency of ~5% in European descent populations, makes the enzyme resistant to cleavage by APC and thus leads to greater levels of the activated form (Bertina et al., 1994). Factor II G20210A (rs1799963), a 3′ untranslated region variant with a minor allele frequency of ~2% in European descent populations, leads to elevated plasma prothrombin levels by increasing the stability of the transcribed mRNA (and, subsequently, greater Factor II synthesis) (Poort et al., 1996; Gehring et al., 2001). Hence, both Factor V Arg506Gln and Factor II G20210A are candidate genetic variants for vascular disease.

Soon after these variants were discovered, investigators sought to test this hypothesis by genotyping DNA collected as part of extant epidemiologic studies. Ridker et al. (1995) determined whether Factor V 506Gln (the allele responsible for the pro-coagulation phenotype) was a risk factor for venous thromboembolism (VTE) in a nested case–control study within the Physicians Health Study. Cases of VTE (n = 121) were identified during an average of 8.6 years of follow-up of ~15,000 physicians, all of whom had provided DNA samples at baseline recruitment. A large number of cohort members with DNA who did not develop VTE (n = 704) were chosen as controls. Cases and controls were compared with respect to carriership of one copy of Factor V 506Gln (the low minor allele frequency precluded assessment of risk associated with 506Gln homozygotes); a strong association was observed (Table 5.1).

In a population-based case–control study, Rosendaal et al. (1997) assessed whether carriership of either Factor V 506Gln or Factor II 20210A is a risk factor for

**Table 5.1.** Prospective study of factor V (FV) Arg506Gln genotypes and risk of venous thromboembolism (adapted from Ridker et al., 1995).

| FV Arg506Gln genotype | Cases (n = 121) | Controls (n = 704) | Odds ratio (95% CI) |
|---|---|---|---|
| Arg/Gln | 11.6% | 6.0% | 2.7 (1.3, 5.6) |
| Arg/Arg | 88.4% | 94.0% | 1.0 (reference) |
| Total | 100.0% | 100.0% | |

*Continued*

**Box 5.1.** Continued.

early-onset myocardial infarction in women. First, incident cases of acute myocardial infarction occurring in women 18–44 years of age were identified from all hospitals in the Seattle–Puget Sound metropolitan region. For comparison, women of the same age living in the same region were identified through random-digit telephone dialing. Cases and controls were recruited into a protocol that included collection of DNA from peripheral white blood cells. The results of the genotyping assays are summarized in Table 5.2, and demonstrated a strong association between these two genetic pro-coagulation factors and the risk of myocardial infarction in young women.

**Table 5.2.** Case–control study of Factor V (FV) Arg506Gln, Factor II (FII) G20210A, and acute myocardial infarction (adapted from Rosendaal *et al.*, 1997).

| FV 506Gln or FII 20210A | Cases (n = 79) | Controls (n = 382) | Odds ratio (95% CI) |
|---|---|---|---|
| Yes | 15.2% | 5.2% | 3.1 (1.5, 6.8) |
| No | 84.8% | 94.8% | 1.0 (reference) |
| Total | 100.0% | 100.0% | |

## 5.3 Complexities of Interpreting Genetic Association Results

Unlike genetic linkage analysis in which results are based on the biological occurrence of recombination during meiosis, the interpretation of genetic association is more complex. There are three basic explanations for an association between an allele and a disease or risk factor: (i) a direct, causal relationship; (ii) an indirect association due to LD; and (iii) a false-positive association (type I error) due to multiple comparisons, deviations of the genetic marker from Hardy–Weinberg equilibrium, and/or population stratification. As with all epidemiologic association studies, there may also be false-negative results, or type II errors as well.

### 5.3.1 Direct, causal relationship

Establishing a causal association between a common genetic variant and disease should be based on meeting the traditional criteria for causality used in epidemiologic research. Koepsell and Weiss (2003) describe a version of these criteria that can be adapted to this genetic context. Ideally, evaluation of causality would be based on randomized controlled clinical trials. Such data are, however, rarely available for genetic variants. Thus, data from observational, non-randomized studies must be used to evaluate causality, as summarized below.

- *Strength and consistency of the association*: How large is the odds ratio, is it statistically significant and how wide is the confidence interval? Further, are the results from different studies and populations consistent, finding similar odds ratios and significant levels?

- *Temporal sequence of events:* Does the suspected cause precede the presence of the disease? Although genotypes are present at birth, the development of symptoms over time and at different ages can provide some useful evidence for this criterion.
- *Dose–response relationship:* This criterion applies when a risk factor is expected to have a continuous quantifiable effect on outcome; that is, an increasing "dose" of exposure to a risk factor is associated with increasing risk of disease. Such a dose relationship might be seen for a risk allele when it is co-dominant, so that it confers a partial effect in heterozygotes and a greater effect in homozygotes.
- *Biological plausibility and consistency with other knowledge:* Genetic variants with known effects on proteins provide important evidence for causality. For example, variants can directly affect the active site of an enzyme or they can affect the stability or protein structure away from an active enzyme site, including resulting in the synthesis of completely inactive protein.
- *Alternative explanations for the association:* Effects such as confounding effect modification, imprecise measure of association with wide confidence intervals, and even different biological mechanisms should be considered when evaluating the evidence for causality.

An example of a known, direct association is illustrated in Box 5.2.

## 5.3.2 Indirect association due to linkage disequilibrium

In most genetic association studies, alleles that are in LD with a disease mutation are identified, rather than the causal allele itself (Manolio, 2010). For example, as described in Section 3.5, tag SNPs that are strongly correlated in a chromosomal region can be used to intentionally and efficiently test for association within and near candidate genes, or across the whole genome. In this way, a possible disease susceptibility allele can be identified, and then followed up by fine-mapping studies and functional characterization of the variant.

---

**Box 5.2. Application: Low-density Lipoprotein Receptor and Coronary Heart Disease**

A well-understood example of clearly functional variants is familial hypercholesterolemia (FH), the low-density lipoprotein receptor (LDLR) gene, and risk of coronary heart disease (Austin *et al.*, 2004). FH is an autosomal genetic disorder characterized by elevated levels of total cholesterol and LDL cholesterol in families. This clinical phenotype is associated with increased risk of coronary heart disease and premature death. The major causes of FH are mutations in LDLR on chromosome 19 that result in significantly increased blood levels of these lipids. There are over 700 mutations in the LDLR gene, the most severe of which are "receptor-negative" mutations that result in no LDLR protein and the most serious clinical phenotype.

---

### 5.3.3 False-positive associations

In addition to direct and indirect genetic associations, investigators must be cautious that an apparently statistically significant association between a genetic marker and a disease may be due to false-positive results.

A major potential source of potential false positives is not controlling for multiple comparisons. As with any epidemiologic association study, type I error (erroneously concluding there is an association when one is not present due to chance) is always a possibility. The traditional significance level of $\alpha = 0.05$ sets this probability at 5%. The more independent comparisons that are made, however, the greater the possibility of this type of error occurring. This is especially important in GWAS, in which a million association tests or more may be performed, one for each marker genotyped. Although a variety of statistical approaches have been proposed to address this problem, the Bonferroni correction (Pearson and Manolio, 2008) remains the standard approach for avoiding false positives owing to multiple comparisons, as described below.

If we define m = number of statistical tests to be performed at $\alpha = 0.05$, and assume that m = 1,000,000 tests in a GWAS, then we would expect to observe 50,000 "statistically significant" SNP associations without adjustment. This is clearly unrealistic and many of these associations will be due to chance. In the Bonferroni adjustment, the significance level is determined by dividing $\alpha$ by the number of tests. For example, in the GWAS with 1 million tests:

$$\alpha = 0.05/m = 0.05/1,000,000 = 0.00000005 = 5 \times 10^{-8}$$

This significance level has become the standard for GWAS such that only p-values $<5 \times 10^{-8}$ are generally considered statistically significant.

It is important to note, however, that the Bonferroni correction may be overly conservative in certain settings, including when the SNP chip being used contains correlated markers. Further, it does not take into account the power of a study (for example a small case–control study), and the resulting number of positive associations that are likely to be true (McCarthy *et al.*, 2008). Thus, less conservative methods such as the false-positive discovery rate (Wacholder *et al.*, 2004) and the Bayesian false-discovery rate (Wakefield, 2007) have been developed to detect "noteworthiness" of observed associations.

A second possible reason for possible false-positive association findings is departure of the genetic marker under study from Hardy–Weinberg equilibrium. This is typically tested using a $\chi^2$ test as described in Section 3.3. Schaid and Jacobsen (1999) have shown that the chance of a false-positive association is inflated if homozygotes for the high-risk allele are more common than predicted under Hardy–Weinberg equilibrium. Conversely, association tests can be too conservative if homozygotes are less frequent than expected. Thus, genetic markers used in a genetic association study should always be tested for Hardy–Weinberg equilibrium, and GWAS often exclude markers that are not found to be in equilibrium (Kanetsky *et al.*, 2009). Because of the large number of markers tested in the context of a GWAS, p-values lower than 0.05 are often used to avoid false-positive tests. Xu *et al.* (2002) have further emphasized the deviations from Hardy–Weinberg equilibrium can be due to several types of systematic genotyping errors, including DNA contamination, lack of blinding to case–control status of study participants, and differential genotyping failure rates for homozygotes and heterozygotes, and thus can be a "hint for genotyping error." To address this concern, the authors recommend a series of practical steps, including blinding to case–control status, including blanks, multiple, and duplicate controls in each plate, and determining the acceptable amount of missing data.

Third, false-positive findings in genetic association studies can be due to population stratification, a form a statistical confounding (Altshuler et al., 2008). Population stratification can be defined as differences in allele frequencies due to ethnic group or ancestry differences between the case group and the control group, resulting in an apparent association that is actually attributable to confounding. Population stratification will be considered in detail in Chapter 6.

### 5.3.4 False-negative associations and power

In the event that a genetic study does not reveal any association with the disease or trait of interest, there is always the possibility of a type II error; that is, there may be an association with one or more genetic variants, but it is not detected in the study. As with false-positive findings, there are several possible explanations that need to be considered. In many genetic association studies, effect sizes are small, and thus large sample sizes are needed for adequate power to detect relationships. If genomic coverage of markers is not sufficient, associated variants may not be detected, especially if there are important rare alleles. These issues are discussed in the context of GWAS in Section 5.4.2 below, and software for power calculations is described in Section 9.2.6. In addition, Wang et al. (2010) provide a concise summary of potential biases in epidemiologic studies of gene–disease associations.

## 5.4 Basics of Genome-wide Association Studies (GWAS)

The National Institute of Health defines a GWAS study as "a study of common genetic variation across the entire human genome designed to identify genetic associations with observable traits" (Pearson and Manolio, 2008). As noted in Section 5.1, GWAS have no prior hypotheses about the variants(s) in the genome that may be associated with the trait of interest. They use high-throughput technologies for genotyping hundreds of thousands or millions of SNPs. In order to have sufficient statistical power to detect the small effect sizes found in most GWAS, very large samples are needed, often obtained through large-scale collaborations (see Section 5.5). Statistical analysis approaches for GWAS emphasize the need to avoid false positives due to multiple hypothesis testing, evaluating possible differences in ancestry between cases and control (population stratification), and the use of discovery and validation phases.

The National Human Genome Research Institute (NHGRI) maintains *A Catalog of Genome-Wide Association Studies* (Hindorff et al., 2009). This catalog, which is continually updated, includes studies that attempt to assay at least 100,000 SNPs, while studies focused only on candidate genes are excluded. The catalog contains studies collected through PubMed literature searches that are conducted weekly, daily news and media reports distributed by the NIH, and by comparing the catalog listings with the GWAS literature in the HuGE Navigator database (Austin et al., 2012).

Based on this catalog, Visscher *et al.* (2012) recently reported that there are more than 2,000 SNPs that have been associated with complex traits and diseases. This includes nearly 500 SNPs reported in the first half of 2011 alone, and thousands of publications since 2007. Although not all investigators agree (McClellan and King, 2010), these authors (Visscher *et al.*, 2012) conclude that GWAS in human populations have led to:

- new discoveries about genes and pathways involved in complex diseases;
- a wealth of new biological insights;
- discoveries with direct clinical utility; and
- facilitation of basic research in human genetics and genomics.

### 5.4.1  GWAS case–control studies

Similar to candidate genes studies, GWAS can be conducted using case–control, cohort, and case–parent trio designs (Pearson and Manolio, 2008). Because a large proportion of GWAS reported to date use a case–control design, we will focus on this study approach first (see Section 5.5 for cohort studies and 5.6 for case–parent trio designs). This design has several important advantages, including that it can be conducted in a short time frame, large numbers of cases and controls can be assembled though large-scale collaborations, and it has the ability to study rare diseases. Case–control studies, however, require several assumptions: cases and controls are drawn from same population; cases are representative of all cases of disease; and genomic and epidemiologic data are collected similarly in cases and controls. Disadvantages include potential bias due to population stratification (confounding); cases are often prevalent and may not include fatal or more severe forms of disease; and, as with all epidemiologic studies, the odds ratio from a case–control study may overstate the true relative risk for common diseases (Pearson and Manolio, 2008). Useful criteria are provided by these authors in the form of "Ten basic questions to ask about a genome-wide association study."

### 5.4.2  Data analysis of GWAS

For the statistical analysis of GWAS data, SNP genotypes are generally coded as allele counts (0, 1, or 2), corresponding to an additive genetic model. Associations between SNPs and disease are then calculated using odds ratios (OR) and 95% confidence intervals, often using logistic regression analysis to adjust for appropriate covariates.

The results are then displayed in the form of a "Manhattan plot," where the "skyscrapers" are significant findings; that is, as shown in Plate 2, chromosomes are displayed on the X axis and p-values on a negative $\log_{10}$ scale for the associations between SNPs and disease are shown on the Y axis. Note that for $p = 0.01$, $-\log_{10} p = -\log_{10}(0.01) = 2$; for $p = 0.001$, $-\log_{10} p = -\log_{10}(0.001) = 3$, etc. Thus, the higher the "skyscraper" is, then the smaller the p-value, and the stronger the evidence for association. In this example from the Wellcome Trust Case Control Consortium (McCarthy *et al.*, 2008), three significant chromosomal regions were found to be associated with type 2 diabetes: the *CDKAL1* gene on chromosome 6, the *TCF7L2* gene on chromosome 10, and the *FTO* gene on chromosome 16.

Quantile–quantile (QQ) plots are another important component of reporting GWAS results (see Section 6.2 for examples). On the X axis of these plots are $-\log_{10}$ of the expected p-values under the null hypothesis of no association, whereas the observed $-\log_{10}$ p-values for each of the SNPs tested in the GWAS are displayed on the Y axis. If no associations are found across the genome, all of these points will fall on or near the 45° line. If confounding resulting from population stratification or cryptic relatedness (unknown genetic relationship among study participants; see Section 9.2.5) is present, many of these points will fall on a line with a slope greater than 1, indicating the presence of a serious bias. If true associations exist, most points should fall on or near the 45°, whereas a few, statistically significant associations are far above the line.

Several special considerations must be taken into account in the analysis of GWAS data. As noted above in Section 5.3.3, significance levels must be adjusted to take into account the large number of genetic association test performed, and the generally accepted significance threshold for GWAS is $p < 5 \times 10^{-8}$. Because of the relatively small effect sizes (ORs often in the range of 1.1–1.3), and multiple comparisons, power for a GWAS based on a single study is generally low (Manolio, 2010). Thus, meta-analyses are often used to combine samples from several studies, increasing the probability of detecting a statistically significant effect (Manolio, 2010). In the setting of meta-analysis, different genotyping platforms are often used, and thus, imputation is used to infer a common set of genotypes for statistical testing and to expand the number of genotypes that can be tested (see Section 9.2.7; de Bakker *et al.*, 2006; Browning, 2008). Finally, as discussed above, potential confounding due to population stratification must also be considered, and this is discussed in detail in Chapter 6.

To demonstrate analysis of GWAS data, and to illustrate that GWAS and candidate gene studies are complementary, two studies of pancreatic cancer are described in Box 5.3.

## 5.5  Large-scale Collaborations: The Cohorts for Heart and Aging Research in Genomic Epidemiology (CHARGE) Consortium

In the last several decades, advances in technology have reduced the costs of genotyping precipitously. Assays for two SNPs, Factor V Leiden and the prothrombin variant, cost US$30 in the late 1990s. Within a decade, genome-wide arrays with hundreds of thousands of SNPs were available for less than US$500. The investment in GWAS by the NIH launched a new era in genetic epidemiology. The Cardiovascular Health Study (CHS), a cohort study of 5,888 older adults from four communities, received one of the grants to a conduct a GWAS. As the genotyping was underway, emails and telephone calls from investigators at other studies with GWAS data inquired whether CHS would be willing to serve as the replication site for the primary GWAS findings of these other studies. Indeed, there were multiple calls from each of the other studies, often one for each major phenotype of interest.

**Box 5.3. Application: Pancreatic Cancer**

**PanScan Consortium**

In 2009, a two-stage GWAS of pancreatic cancer was published by the PanScan Consortium of 12 prospective and nine case–control studies (Amundadottir *et al.*, 2009).

In stage 1 of the study, cases with pancreatic cancer were obtained from 12 prospective studies and one case–control study. The case definition was adenocarcinoma of the exocrine pancreas (non-exocrine tumors of the pancreas were excluded), and controls were matched on year of birth, sex, race, ethnicity and DNA sample type. A total of 1,770 incident cases were identified with one matched control per case. In addition, 368 cases from the Mayo Clinic case–control study provided informed consent and blood for this stage of the analysis, and 345 clinic controls were frequency matched on age, race, sex, and residence area. Either blood or buccal cells had been collected from the study participants for DNA extraction and genotyping. Stage 2 of the study for replication consisted of participants from eight case–control studies, comprising 2,457 cases and 2,654 controls.

The online methods section of the paper, and the supplementary tables and figures, describe the genotyping, quality control, and statistical analysis approaches. A total of 4,063 DNA samples, representing 3,932 individuals, and 129 that were analyzed in duplicate, were selected for the study. The Human Hap 500 Infinium Assay (Illumina) was used and 561,466 SNP genotypes were attempted. Samples with less than 98% complete rates were excluded after a second attempt at genotyping. Following quality-control procedures, including cluster plots, 558,542 SNPs across the genome were available for analysis.

For the statistical analysis, SNP genotypes were coded as allele minor counts (0, 1, or 2), corresponding to an additive genetic model. Associations between SNP and pancreatic cancer were assessed using logistic regression analysis adjusted for age, sex, study, study arm (intervention versus observation for the Women's Health Initiative), ancestry, and genetic structure. First, the data for each study were analyzed separately, then pooled across studies and tested for heterogeneity of results. The QQ plot of observed versus expected p-values did not give evidence for systematic error due to population structure (data not shown).

In stage 1, the Manhattan plot shows an association between pancreatic cancer and a cluster of SNPs on chromosome 9 (Plate 3). A regional plot of that area of chromosome 9 (Plate 4) demonstrates that two of the strongest signals were for a base pair change from T to C for marker rs505922 and a C to T change for rs630014 in the ABO blood group gene. The odds ratios for these markers are shown in Table 5.3 for stages 1 and 2 of the study. For rs505922, the C allele was associated with increased risk of pancreatic cancer in both stages, and these results were similar for European individuals in the study and for all ethnic groups combined (data not shown). In contrast, the rs630014 marker was associated with decreased risk at both stages.

Plate 4 further shows that these two SNPs are in LD with each other ($r^2 = 0.52$ based on HapMap data and 0.40 in PanScan data) and both are located within a haplotype block that encompasses the promoter and introns 1 and 2 of the ABO gene.

The authors of this study conclude that genetic variation at the ABO locus on chromosome 9q34 may influence risk of pancreatic carcinogenesis. In particular, the "protective" T allele for the rs505922 SNP is in complete LD ($r^2 = 1$) with the O

*Continued*

M.A. Austin *et al.*

**Box 5.3.** Continued.

**Table 5.3.** Association of SNPs on chromosome 9 with risk of pancreatic cancer (adapted from Amundadottir *et al.*, 2009).

| SNP | p-value | Odds ratio (95% confidence interval) | |
|---|---|---|---|
| | | Heterozygous | Homozygous |
| rs505922 (T > C) | | | |
|     Stage 1 | $2.5 \times 10^{-6}$ | 1.3 (1.1, 1.4) | 1.6 (1.3, 1.9) |
|     Stage 2 | $2.1 \times 10^{-3}$ | 1.2 (1.1, 1.3) | 1.3 (1.1, 1.6) |
| rs630014 (C > T) | | | |
|     Stage 1 | $4.3 \times 10^{-5}$ | 0.8 (0.8, 0.9) | 0.7 (0.6, 0.8) |
|     Stage 2 | $5.8 \times 10^{-4}$ | 0.9 (0.8, 0.9) | 0.7 (0.6, 0.9) |

allele of the ABO locus, and implies that the A and B alleles could increase risk. In fact, studies from the 1950s and 1960 found associations between the ABO blood groups and risk of gastrointestinal cancer, and ABO antigen expression has been found to altered in pancreatic cancers compared with normal pancreatic cells. Thus, these findings "could contribute to improvements in risk stratification, prevention, early detection and therapeutic approaches..." to this lethal cancer (Amundadottir *et al.*, 2009).

## Nurses' Health Study and Health Professionals Follow-up Study

At approximately the same time as the GWAS described above, results were published from a combined analysis of data from the Nurses' Health Study (NHS) and the Health Professionals Follow-up Study (NPFS) on the ABO blood group type and risk of pancreatic cancer (Wolpin *et al.*, 2009). These findings illustrate how GWAS and candidate gene studies are complementary, and can provide confirmatory evidence for associations between genetic variants and risk of complex diseases.

The NHS began in 1976 and consists of a cohort of 77,360 female nurses who provide biennial updates on lifestyle, medical history, and diet. The HPFS began in 1986 and includes 30,143 male dentists, veterinarians, pharmacists, optometrists, osteopathic physicians, and podiatrists who also provide biennial questionnaire updates. In a 1996 questionnaire, study participants self-reported ABO blood group as A, B, AB, O, or unknown, and laboratory confirmation was obtained on 98 subjects. Based on next-of-kin reports, hospital records, and the National Death Index, a total of 316 pancreatic cancer cases were identified, 96% of which were histologically confirmed.

The results of the Cox proportional hazards analysis are summarized in Table 5.4 and the strongest association was seen with the B blood type. When all non-O blood groups were combined, the hazard ratio was 1.4 (95% confidence interval 1.1, 1.8) and the population-attributable fraction was 17%.

By combining data from both cohorts, 927,995 person-years of follow-up were observed. The resulting age-adjusted incidence rates of pancreatic cancer were lowest for the O blood type (27/100,000 person-years), higher for A and AB blood types (36 and 41/100,000 person-years, respectively), and highest for B blood type (46/100,000 person-years). Similar trends were also seen for cumulative incidence.

*Continued*

**Box 5.3.** Continued.

These results, based on self-reported ABO blood types, concur with the GWAS SNP results described above, both demonstrating that the O blood type is related to decreased risk of pancreatic cancer compared with A, B, and AB blood types. These confirmatory findings then provide a strong basis for further studies to elucidate the biological mechanisms involved.

**Table 5.4.** Adjusted hazard ratios for the association of ABO blood types and risk of pancreatic cancer, compared with type O (adapted from Wolpin *et al.*, 2009).

| Study | A blood type | AB blood type | B blood type |
|---|---|---|---|
| NHS | 1.3 | 1.6 | 1.7 |
| HPFS | 1.5 | 1.4 | 1.8 |
| Total (95% confidence interval) | 1.3 (1.0, 1.7) | 1.5 (1.0, 2.2) | 1.7 (1.3, 2.4) |

In the 1980s, the National Heart Lung and Blood Institute (NHLBI) had launched several cohort studies that turned out to be genealogically related. Though the participants differed in their age at recruitment, one study often used or borrowed from another study some of the methods to assess novel and traditional risk factors and outcomes. For instance, CHS, a study in older adults, adapted the cardiac outcome criteria from the Atherosclerosis Risk in Communities Study (ARIC), a study of about 16,000 middle-aged adults. Despite their large sample sizes, however, these cohort studies were individually too small to detect effect sizes – relative risks in the range of 1.2–1.3 – that were commonly seen in GWAS (Hindorff *et al.*, 2009). Collaboration would be essential to the discovery and replication of genetic associations. Each cohort study had its own administrative structure and set of investigators. Although investigators from several cohorts had occasionally collaborated, there was no precedent for a consortium of cardiovascular epidemiology cohorts in the USA or internationally. In late 2007, nonetheless, it became clear that, because all cohorts had GWAS data, a prospective population-based design, and a large number of phenotypes assessed by similar data-collection methods, a cohort-level collaboration would be efficient and facilitate a series of prospectively planned joint analyses.

## 5.5.1 The CHARGE Consortium

The CHARGE Consortium first emerged as an investigator-initiated effort from a series of biweekly conference calls that began in June 2007 among the investigators from several large cohort studies. The criteria for membership were a cohort study with cardiovascular or aging phenotypes and GWAS data available by early 2008.

The original five CHARGE cohorts were the Age, Gene/Environment Susceptibility (AGES)–Reykjavik Study, ARIC, CHS, the Framingham Heart Study (FHS), and the Rotterdam Study (RS). The parent studies still review and approve all paper proposals and manuscripts that emerge from CHARGE.

## 5.5.2 CHARGE goals and organization

The primary aim is the conduct of high-quality analyses that produce timely, reliable, and valid findings across multiple cardiovascular and aging-related phenotypes (Psaty *et al.*, 2009). The organizational structure, which is simple, includes a Research Steering Committee (RSC), an Analysis Committee, a Genotyping Committee, and approximately 35 phenotype-specific Working Groups. The RSC, which has two representatives from each cohort, is responsible for establishing the other committees, for nominating working group members, and for developing general guidelines for collaboration, authorship, sharing of results, publication, and timely participation. The Analysis Committee develops guidelines that the working groups are encouraged to adopt or adapt, and the Genotyping Committee coordinates consortium-wide genotyping. The RSC recommendations are advisory, and the primary decision-making authority rests with the phenotype-specific working groups. CHARGE consortium agreements and data-sharing recommendations are available on the public website (Cohorts for Heart and Aging Research in Genetic Epidemiology (CHARGE) Consortium, 2012).

## 5.5.3 Genome-wide genotyping methods

The CHARGE consortium was developed after each cohort study had already contracted for their genotyping platforms. Indeed, the original five cohorts used four different platforms, which have fewer than about 60,000 SNPs in common. To maximize the availability of comparable genetic data and coverage of the genome, each cohort used recently developed methods to impute genotypes for Europeans, European Americans, and African Americans.

## 5.5.4 Design of CHARGE analyses

For many investigators, a two-stage design – with discovery followed by replication – made the most sense. That structure is standard in science. The original CHS design called for a two-stage approach: a limited set of genotypes from the discovery phase would be brought forward for genotyping in the second stage. The primary advantage of this two-stage approach is a reduction in the genotyping costs at the second stage. But from the outset, all the CHARGE cohorts already had GWAS data, so the two-stage approach could not reduce genotyping costs. Indeed, the most powerful method of identifying genuine genetic associations is an analysis that includes all participants from all of the cohorts. The biostatisticians on the Analysis Committee favored the method of meta-analysis, which is as statistically efficient as a cohort-adjusted pooled analysis of individual-level data. Indeed, the committee's early recommendation to use meta-analysis rather than a two-stage discovery–replication design proved to be a powerful social force in promoting collaboration within each working group. This approach avoided the scientific class system that values discovery over replication: each cohort participated more or less equally in a joint meta-analysis. The coordinated prospectively planned meta-analyses of the CHARGE consortium also avoided the practical and legal complexity of international individual-level data sharing among what would turn out to be scores of studies.

## 5.5.5 Phenotype working groups

The wide range of health-related phenotypes measured in these large population-based cohort studies quickly spawned several dozen phenotype-specific working groups. The working groups standardize phenotypes across the studies, decide whether to include other non-member studies with similar phenotypes, and formulate analysis plans. Investigators from each cohort, who know their data well, conduct the association analyses, which are then combined across studies by meta-analysis. The unit of work is the manuscript, and for each project, the phenotype working groups establish plans for authorship, review results, compose manuscripts, and decide on follow-up genotyping or functional work. For each manuscript, the working-group investigators prospectively establish pre-specified plans for analysis and timelines for participation. Working group members agree not to share the GWAS findings with outside groups without the permission of the members who generated the data. Transparency, disclosure, and communications about all collaborations, additional follow-up experiments, or efforts to obtain additional funding have been essential to developing, ensuring, and maintaining trust within each of the consortium's working groups. Many CHARGE working groups have already engaged investigators from non-member studies as collaborators. Collaborating non-member studies either agree to the overall CHARGE principles, or the CHARGE working group develops and negotiates a new CHARGE-compatible agreement with the non-member studies or consortia.

## 5.5.6 Analysis methods

From the start, the CHARGE Analysis Committee developed a set of general plans as guidelines for all working groups. The issues include quality control of genotype data, decisions about what results to share across cohorts, formats for sharing data, strand alignments, coding of alleles, choice of covariates for adjustments, detection of and correction for population structure, stratification of analyses by race/ethnicity, within-study phenotype analysis plans, between-study meta-analysis methods, gene-by-environment analyses, and the importance of written analysis plans prior to sharing the results. For traits that are comparable across studies, the within-study results are combined according to the pre-specified plan, usually by fixed-effects meta-analysis to obtain summary estimates of the effect size, the standard error, the confidence interval, and the p-value. The task of meta-analysis has been shared among all the cohorts. The goal of the Analysis Committee's recommendations was to provide a flexible plan that could be adapted or adopted by working groups. For each stage in the analysis, there are several valid options available. For example, to address multiple testing, the CHARGE Analysis Committee recommends pre-specifying a fixed p-value threshold, but the decision about the exact threshold to use is left up to the working groups. The GWAS experiences of the Analysis Committee, shared across the working groups, simplified the effort for many of the phenotype-specific working groups.

### 5.5.7 Productivity

CHARGE was formed in February 2008, and all cohorts had at least some GWAS data available by June 2008. Since then, CHARGE investigators have published more than 140 papers, and more than 75 are main or primary GWAS papers published or in press. Many CHARGE publications have appeared in high-impact journals, including 24 in *Nature Genetics*, four in *Nature*, two in *JAMA*, two in the *Lancet*, and one in the *New England Journal of Medicine*. The list of CHARGE publications appears at: http://web.chargeconsortium.com/.

### 5.5.8 Collaborations with non-CHARGE studies and other consortia

Of about 35 active working groups, eight collaborate with 20 or more studies. Several patterns have emerged in the evolution of consortia. First, for some phenotypes such as glucose and lipids, phenotype-specific GWAS consortia had already existed when CHARGE was formed, and the relevant CHARGE Working Groups have largely participated in these international efforts such as MAGIC and Global Lipids (Dupuis *et al.*, 2010; Saxena *et al.*, 2010). A second pattern has become apparent for phenotypes such as blood pressure, QT interval, pulmonary function, and red-cell traits. For instance, as the CHARGE Blood Pressure Working Group was finalizing its papers, investigators became aware of Global BPgen, another large consortium with GWAS data on blood pressure. Investigators from the two consortia shared data on high-signal markers and submitted companion papers that were published together in *Nature Genetics* (Levy *et al.*, 2009; Newton-Cheh *et al.*, 2009). Both consortia then began collaboration on full inter-consortia meta-analyses, which resulted in the discovery of 16 novel loci, published in *Nature* (Ehret *et al.*, 2011).

### 5.5.9 Working-group model as innovation

The working-group model emerged in CHS, where several senior investigators invited junior investigators from CHS and non-CHS institutions to participate in epidemiologic research related to renal impairment and cardiovascular disease. By sharing the CHS data and making it widely available to young investigators, the CHS scientists mentored a whole generation of new investigators, who gained confidence and experience as leaders of collaborative publications. Young scientists were encouraged to serve as "champions." From the start, CHARGE adopted both the CHS working group model and the focus on young investigators. About half of the first authors of CHARGE publications have been students, post-doctoral fellows, or junior faculty. In the setting of CHARGE, moreover, the working-group model helped over time to establish multi-institutional, multi-study, international, and interdisciplinary "virtual laboratories" populated both by senior scientists and by eager well-trained young investigators. Indeed, some of these working groups have served as the setting for additional grant applications and even for K-award applications from young investigators.

### 5.5.10   A new era of consortia

The genotyping technologies have served as a powerful force for collaboration among studies, and CHARGE is simply one example of a major trend in epidemiological studies. Many GWAS consortia have formed around specific phenotypes such as diabetes or lipids. Although the CHARGE Consortium uses the prospective cohort study design rather than the phenotype as its organizing principle, its working groups often function as independent consortia. Other large-scale collaborations such as the FDA Sentinel initiative (Behrman *et al.*, 2011) have adopted a distributed data model similar to the one used on CHARGE. The alternative model, the assembly of data from individual studies into a single large dataset, is used, for instance, by the Emerging Risk Factor Consortium (Emerging Risk Factors Collaboration *et al.*, 2010).

### 5.5.11   CHARGE: past, present, and future

The CHARGE Consortium, which takes advantage of the hundreds of millions of dollars invested in these cohort studies, represents an innovative model of investigator-initiated collaborative research to identify genetic loci associated with a variety of cardiovascular and aging phenotypes. The approach – the within-study analysis followed by a between-study meta-analysis – avoids the human subject issues associated with individual-level data sharing among studies from multiple studies and nations. Phenotype experts who know the studies and the data well are responsible for phenotype standardization across cohorts, and the Analysis Committee provides consortium-wide guidance on a variety of issues. An infra-structure grant has provided organizational support for a Coordinating Center, support for two meetings per year, and support for junior-investigator exchanges between CHARGE cohorts. Even though the grant applications that funded the original single-study genome-wide genotyping effort have ended, the cohorts have recently committed to genotyping their participants with the Illumina Exome Chip, a genotyping array that has about 250,000 rare variants discovered by exome sequencing. With the prospect of these new data,

CHARGE investigators are actively pursuing new grant applications to support their working groups or exome-chip data analysis in the consortium more broadly. The prospect of whole-genome sequencing of participants in these well-phenotyped cohorts has excited the interest of investigators. There is, however, no commitment from the NIH to provide ongoing support for an effort such as the CHARGE consortium. At this time, CHARGE remains a fragile entity that depends on successful investigator-initiated applications to maintain its high level of productivity.

### 5.5.12 Facilitating large-scale collaborations

The CHARGE Consortium illustrates that GWAS consortia have been successful owing to a variety of timely developments. These include: innovations in genomic technology, availability of DNA samples and comprehensive epidemiologic data from large population-based studies, computational advances in the management of massive datasets and new statistical approaches, the need for unprecedented samples sizes for sufficient statistical power, the need for replication in different populations, internet-based communication, and data sharing among hundreds of collaborating investigators, as well as NIH policies requiring data sharing and encouraging data harmonization of phenotypes.

## 5.6 Case–Parent Trio Designs in GWAS

The basics of this study design approach and the transmission disequilibrium test (TDT) were described in Section 4.2.2. In the context of GWAS, a major advantage of this approach is that it avoids potential bias due to population stratification. Other advantages include that it allows for quality control through checking Mendelian inheritance of markers, it does not require phenotype data for parents, it allows for determination of phase for haplotypes, and it may be logistically simpler for studies of childhood diseases (Pearson and Manolio, 2008). The uses of TDT and other family-based designs in GWAS have recently been reviewed by Ott *et al.* (2011).

## 5.7 Heritability and Allelic Architecture of Complex Traits

### 5.7.1 Missing heritability in GWAS

As described in Section 5.4, more than 2,000 SNPs have been associated with complex traits and diseases to date based on GWAS (Visscher *et al.*, 2012). However, as Manolio *et al.* (2009) report, "... it is now clear that common risk variants fail to explain the vast majority of genetic heritability for many human diseases ... " This debate has been described as whether the "glass is half full or half empty" (D. Nickerson, personal communication); that is, half full because thousands of SNP–disease associations have been found, or half empty because most of the heritability of diseases is not explained by these associations.

Manolio and colleagues (2009) further note that this "missing heritability" may take different forms across common, complex diseases because of variation in their "allelic architecture": the number of alleles that impact disease predisposition, their effect sizes, and their frequencies (Pritchard and Cox, 2002). For example, for some diseases, heritability may be explained by a small number of common variants with large effects, whereas for other diseases there may be a large number of variants each with a small effect. Further, there may be susceptibility genes with common variants that also contain rare variants with larger effects, and associations may differ by environment and/or by ethnic group.

In Fig. 5.1, these authors illustrate the feasibility of identifying genetic variants for disease by allele frequency (X axis) and by effect size (Y axis). The "common disease/ common variant" hypothesis (Risch and Merikangas, 1996) addresses relatively common alleles with a minor allele frequency (MAF) of 0.05 or greater, but with small effects sizes (ORs of 1.1–1.5), shown in the bottom right of the graph. These are the types of variants that are generally found in GWAS. In contrast, very rare Mendelian diseases are often caused by alleles with large effect sizes that can be detected using exome sequencing (Ng *et al.*, 2010b; Bamshad *et al.*, 2011), shown in the upper left of the graph. However, it is possible that at least some of the "missing heritability" for common diseases is attributable to relatively low frequency variants with modest effect sizes (0.01 < MAF < 0.05, ORs > 1.5), shown in the center of the graph. These types of variants are the focus of many ongoing studies using next-generation sequencing technology, facilitated by the data being generated by the 1,000 Genomes Project (see Chapters 4 and 9). Other possible explanations for such missing heritability are considered in Box 5.4, using human height as an example.

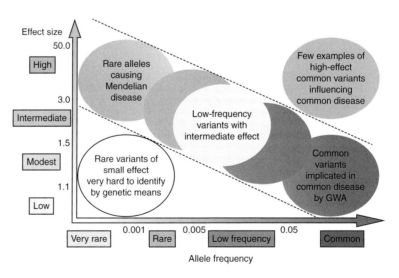

**Fig. 5.1.** Feasibility of identifying genetic variants by risk allele frequency and strength of genetic effect (odds ratio) (reprinted with permission from Manolio *et al.*, 2009).

M.A. Austin *et al.*

**Box 5.4. Application: Height**

**Historical context**

Scientists have been interested in genetic influences on human height for more than 100 years, and it was one of the first traits to be studied using the GWAS approach. Based on data that he collected about more than 1,000 adult children and their parents, Francis Galton wrote, "For every unit that the stature of any group of men of the same height deviates upwards or downwards from the level of mediocrity [the mean] their brothers will on average deviate only two thirds of a unit, their sons one third, their nephews two ninths and the grandsons one ninth" (Galton, 1886). In 1903, Karl Pearson developed a regression for the relationship between a son's stature and his father's (Pearson and Lee, 1903):

Son's stature (inches) = 33.73 + 0.516 (father's stature)

Long before the common disease/common variant hypothesis had been described, R.A. Fisher (1918) proposed that, "The simplest hypothesis is that such features as stature are determined by a large number of Mendelian factors, and that the large variance among children of the same parents is due to the segregation of those factors in respect to which the parents are heterozygous."

**Missing heritability of height from early GWAS**

In May 2008, three papers were published in the same issue of *Nature Genetics* describing associations between genetic variants and height using GWAS approaches (Gudbjartsson *et al.*, 2008; Lettre *et al.*, 2008; Weedon *et al.*, 2008). As shown in Table 5.5, these studies combined included nearly 69,000 participants. Although many associated genetic variants were found, these only explained a small proportion of the variation in human height in these samples.

In this section, we will consider three possibilities for the "missing heritability" of height based on GWAS:

1. Are effect sizes too small to be detected even in GWAS with large sample sizes?
2. Are the identified loci biologically relevant?
3. Is the traditional $h^2$ estimate of 0.80 (Visscher, 2008) too high?

Note that the possible roles of epistasis and gene–environment interaction are considered in Section 2.3.3.

**Table 5.5.** GWAS of height published in May, 2008.

| Study | Sample size | Number of associated loci | Population variability explained |
|---|---|---|---|
| Lettre *et al.*, 2008 | 15,821 | 12 | 2% |
| Weedon *et al.*, 2008 | 13,665 | 20 | 3% |
| Gudbjartsson *et al.*, 2008 | 39,510 | 27 | 3.7% |

*Continued*

**Box 5.4.** Continued.

## Effect sizes

In July, 2010, two papers also published in *Nature Genetics* began to reveal "Hints of hidden heritability in GWAS" and to address the possibility that the missing genetic variance is "hidden" below the stringent threshold of $5 \times 10^{-8}$ for statistical significance used in GWAS because of small effect sizes (Gibson, 2010).

Using a quantitative genetic approach, Yang *et al.* (2010) analyzed a set of 3,925 unrelated individuals for the association of 294,831 SNPs across the genome with height. Instead of testing each SNP individually, they used a linear regression model that fits all SNPs simultaneously, and accounted for 45% of the variance in height. By further correcting for imperfect linkage disequilibrium between causal variants and the genotyped SNPs, possibly because the causal variants have lower MAF than the genotyped SNPs, this estimate increased even further.

In the second paper, Park *et al.* (2010) propose a method to estimate, on the basis of available GWAS data, the number of additional loci with common variants that can be expected to be found and the sample sizes needed to detect these. Based on the 54 loci detected in the three GWAS of height above, they estimate that 201 SNPs exist for height (95% confidence interval 75, 494) with similar effect sizes and that more than 100,000 study subjects would be needed to detect these.

## Biological relevance

Remarkably, a study on this order of magnitude was published within a few months. In a meta-analysis of 183,727 individuals studying nearly 3,000,000 SNPs, Lango Allen *et al.* (2010) reported associations with 180 SNPs meeting the $5 \times 10^{-8}$ threshold for statistical significance that explained approximately 10% of the phenotypic variance in adult height. Importantly, these loci are enriched for genes in connected biological pathways, with the likely causal gene often located near the most strongly associated variants. The top ten key words for these genes were: growth, kinase, factor, transcription, signaling, binding, differentiation, development, insulin, and bone (Lango Allan *et al.*, 2010). Further, 19 of these loci had multiple independently related variants, suggesting allelic heterogeneity for these associated genes. The authors conclude that "GWA studies can identify large numbers of loci that implicate biologically relevant genes and pathways."

## Traditional estimates of heritability too high

Although lower estimates have been reported, the heritability of height is approximately 0.80, indicating that approximately 80% of the variation in height among individuals is due to genetic influences (Silventoinen, 2003). Most of these estimates have, however, been reported from twin studies, and as described in Chapter 2, there are many possible biases that can influence such estimates.

Traditional heritability estimates are based on the *expected* proportion of shared alleles between relatives. For twin studies, it is assumed that dizygous (DZ) twins share ½ of alleles on *average*, whereas monozygous (MZ) pairs share all alleles. Visscher *et al.* (2006) have described an alternative approach using genome-wide data that estimates shared genetic variance based on the *observed* proportion of the genome that is shared identical by descent (IBD), and have used this method to estimate heritability of height.

*Continued*

M.A. Austin *et al.*

**Box 5.4.** Continued.

In this analysis, the authors used 4,401 quasi-independent full-sibling pairs from two cohorts of Australian twins and their siblings, and the number of available genetic markers ranged from 201 to 1,717. IBD sharing (see Chapter 3) was estimated at 1 cM (centiMorgan) intervals and averaged over the whole genome for each subject. Genome-wide heritability estimates can then be determined as follows:

For $i = 1, \ldots n$ sib pairs with heights $(Y_{i1}, Y_{i2})$:

$\Pi_i$ = genome-wide IBD sharing = $\frac{1}{2}\Pi^p + \frac{1}{2}\Pi^m$
where p = paternal, m = maternal contributions.

Using Haseman–Elston regression:

$(Y_{i1} - Y_{i2})^2 = \alpha + \beta\Pi_i$
$\beta = -2\sigma_A^2$ (assuming parents are not inbred)

The estimated heritability is then:

$h^2 = -\hat{\beta}/2s_P^2 = 2s_A^2/2s_P^2 = s_A^2/s_P^2$

where $s_A^2$ is estimated additive genetic variance and $s_P^2$ is estimated total phenotypic variance of height.

Using this approach, heritability of height was confirmed to be 80%, in both adolescents and adults from this sample, as shown in Table 5.6.

Thus, at least based on the analytic approach using genome data, the traditional estimates of the heritability of height do not appear to be overestimated.

## Summary

As described in this section, the debate about the reasons for the "missing heritability" in GWAS studies is likely to continue. It is also important, however, to keep the controversy in perspective. As Manolio and colleagues note (2009), "Explaining missing heritability is ... however intellectually satisfying ... a means to an end. The ultimate goal of this line of research ... is to improve understanding of human physiology and disease etiology so that more effective means of diagnosis, treatment and prevention can be developed."

**Table 5.6.** Maximum likelihood estimates of heritability of height from genome-wide IBD sharing between sib pairs (adapted from Visscher *et al.*, 2006).

| Sample | Heritability (95% confidence interval) | |
|---|---|---|
| Adolescents (N = 931) | 0.80 | (0.00, 0.90) |
| Adults (N = 2,444) | 0.80 | (0.43, 0.86) |
| Combined sample | 0.80 | (0.46, 0.85) |

## 5.8  Study Designs and Statistical Analysis of DNA Sequencing Data

As noted in Section 3.6, unlike most genome-wide SNP chips that are designed primarily to detect common variation, DNA sequencing data can be used to detect associations of rare genetic variants with disease. These types of data require specific study design strategies for common and rare diseases, and different statistical analysis approaches. In particular, sequencing allows the direct identification of causal variants, rather than relying on LD patterns between common markers and disease mutations used in most GWAS (Kiezun *et al.*, 2012).

### 5.8.1 Study designs for rare genetic variants

Two distinct study designs, described below, have been proposed as strategies for identifying rare genetic variants underlying disease susceptibility (Cirulli and Goldstein, 2010; Bamshad *et al.*, 2011).

#### *Sequencing relatives in families with multiple affected individuals*

Although somewhat counter-intuitive, this strategy often involves sequencing the distantly related, affected, family members. This is because the more distantly related these family members are, the fewer genetic variants they will share. But, assuming the disease of interest is caused by the same variant in both relatives, they should share that causal variant. First cousins, for example, share approximately 1/8 of their genomes IBD. However, when using this strategy, distant relatives will still share too much of their genomes to allow simple identification of the causal variants. Thus, the associated variants need to be screened or "filtered" based on function, allele frequency, and/or the type of gene affected. Another tactic for narrowing the variants of interest is to use evidence of modest linkage based on LOD score analysis (Cirulli and Goldstein, 2010). Box 4.3 in Chapter 4 describes how these approaches are being used to investigate genetic influences on prostate cancer.

Using a type of case–parent trio design (Section 4.2.2), sequencing affected offspring and their unaffected parents can also be used to identify *de novo* mutations for disease (Bamshad *et al.*, 2011). This approach and its application to studies of autism spectrum disorders are described in Section 8.3 and Box 8.2.

Following the first "proof of concept" study demonstrating that whole-exome sequencing could be used to identify a known causal mutation for a rare, Mendelian disease (Freeman–Sheldon syndrome) (Ng *et al.*, 2009), the unknown cause of another rare Mendelian disease, Miller syndrome, was identified by performing whole-exome sequencing in four cases from three families and eight controls (Ng *et al.*, 2010a). Building on these discoveries, exome sequencing has been shown to be a successful approach for understanding several unsolved Mendelian diseases (Ng *et al.*, 2010b). Large-scale studies such as the NHBLI Grand Opportunities Exome Sequencing Project (ESP) (2012) are now applying exome sequencing technology to common, complex diseases such as heart, lung, and blood disorders (Tennessen *et al.*, 2012).

#### *Extreme trait sequencing*

The second strategy, which is especially well suited for quantitative traits, is to sequence a small number of carefully selected study participants from one or both ends of the phenotype distribution (Cirulli and Goldstein, 2010). The frequency of alleles contributing to disease susceptibility is expected to be enriched in these extremes of the distribution, and thus can be identified based on a relatively modest number of cases and controls.

The potential for this strategy was demonstrated in an early study of high-density lipoprotein (HDL) cholesterol (Cohen *et al.*, 2004). In this study, three candidate genes were sequenced in only 38 individuals from the upper and lower 5% of the HDL cholesterol distribution. The results demonstrated that rare alleles had significant effects on low HDL cholesterol, a major risk factor for coronary heart disease. In one of the first findings from the NHLBI ESP project, extreme phenotypes were used to determine that variants in the *DCTN4* gene, which encodes a dynactin protein, is associated with chronic *Pseudomonas aeruginosa* infection among individuals with cystic fibrosis (Emond *et al.*, 2012). Such infections are related to reduced lung function and shorter mean survival. In this study, 43 individuals with an early age of onset for the infection were compared with 48 of the oldest individuals who did not have a chronic infection, and the presence of one or more missense mutations in the *DCTN4* gene was associated with early age at onset of the infection (hazard ratio = 1.9, P = 0.004). The authors indicate that the success of this exome sequencing study of a complex trait with a small sample size is attributable to the well-matched extremes, the large effect size of the gene, and the relatively high combined MAF (0.065) for the rare variants examined. However, initial analyses based on deep sequencing of rare coding variation of 2,440 individuals from the ESP project demonstrate that large sample sizes will be needed for sufficient power in association studies of rare variants with most complex diseases (Tennessen *et al.*, 2012).

### 5.8.2 Methods for detecting association with rare variants

Statistical methods for discovering association of rare genetic variants with disease risk are developing rapidly. These approaches are fundamentally different from statistics used for association with common genetic variants (Kiezun *et al.*, 2012). This is because rare variants must be combined in a gene, a biological pathway, or a regulatory region ("unit based"), rather than testing individual variants, in order to increase inherent low statistical power. Further, population genetic information and functional data can be added to the analysis. Examples of three such "burden tests" are summarized below (Kiezun *et al.*, 2012):

- Combined Multivariate and Collapsing (CMC) (Li and Leal, 2008). This method jointly assesses the role of rare and common variants by applying a multivariate test on the collapsed rare variants and a traditional regression-based association for the uncollapsed common variants.
- Weighted Sum Statistic (WSS) (Madsen and Browning, 2009). In this approach, mutations are grouped according to function (gene) and each individual is given a score of mutation counts, weighted by the inverse of the binomial variance. A rank sum test is used to compare case and control groups. This method accentuates rare mutations in the controls and insures that common mutations do not dominate the test.
- C-alpha Test Statistic (Neale *et al.*, 2011). To take into account possible differences in the directionality of effects (risk or protective) of mutation being tested, this test is designed to maintain power when target mutation effects are in opposite directions in the same genetic region.

Similar to the analysis of data from GWAS studies, multiple comparisons, statistical power, replication, and population stratification must all be considered in the analysis of exome sequencing data (Emond *et al.*, 2012; Kiezun *et al.*, 2012). For example, assuming one test per gene, exome sequencing studies involve approximately 20,000 independent association tests. Using a Bonferroni correction, a significance level of 0.05 corresponds to a p-value threshold of $2.5 \times 10^{-6}$ per gene.

## 5.9  Conclusion

Building on the "common disease/common variant" hypothesis described in the 1990s, genetic association studies of unrelated individuals have been successful in identifying susceptibility genes for complex diseases, using both candidate gene and genome-wide approaches. These approaches are complementary and can use a variety of traditional epidemiologic study designs. However, in contrast to linkage analysis, interpretation of genetic association results must be undertaken with caution, taking into consideration many possible sources of bias. The CHARGE Consortium is an example of an effective and productive GWAS collaboration that has used innovations in genomic technology, availability of DNA samples and comprehensive epidemiologic data from large population-based studies, and computational advances and new statistical approaches to advance our understanding of genetic susceptibility to cardiovascular diseases and risk factor.

More recently, the alternative "common disease/rare variant" hypothesis, combined with rapid advances in DNA sequencing, is bringing new insights to understanding common diseases through genetic association studies of rare variants and disease.

## Acknowledgments

Research in Section 5.5 was supported in part by grants HL078888, HL080295, HL085251, HL087652, HL103612, and HL105756 from the National Heart, Lung, and Blood Institute. The content is solely the responsibility of the authors and does not necessarily represent the official views of the National Heart, Lung, and Blood Institute or the National Institutes of Health. The authors would like to thank Dr Susan Heckbert for content in Section 5.4.2 and Dr Bruce Weir for content in Box 5.4.

## Further Reading

Bamshad, M.J., Ng, S.B., Bigham, A.W., Tabor, H.K., Emond, M.J., Nickerson, D.A. and Shendure J. (2011) Exome sequencing as a tool for Mendelian disease gene discovery. *Nature Reviews Genetics* 12, 745–755.

Cirulli, E.T. and Goldstein, D.B. (2010) Uncovering the roles of rare variants in common disease through whole-genome sequencing. *Nature Reviews Genetics* 11, 415–425.

Kiezun, A., Garilmella, K., Do, R., Stitziel, N.O., Neale, B.M., McLaren, P.J., *et al.* (2012) Exome sequencing and the genetic basis of complex traits. *Nature Genetics* 44, 623–629.

Manolio, T.A. (2010) Genomewide association studies and assessment of the risk of disease. *New England Journal of Medicine* 363, 166–176.

Pearson, T.A. and Manolio, T.A. (2008) How to interpret a genome-wide association study. *JAMA* 299, 1335–1344.

# References

Altshuler, D., Daly, M.J. and Lander, E.S. (2008) Genetic mapping in human disease. *Science* 322, 881–888.

Amundadottir, L., Kraft, P., Stolzenberg-Solomon, R.Z., Fuchs, C.S., Petersen, G.M., Arslan, A.A., *et al.* (2009) Genome-wide association study identifies variants in the ABO locus associated with susceptibility to pancreatic cancer. *Nature Genetics* 41, 986–990.

Austin, M.A., Hutter, C.M., Zimmern, R.L. and Humphries, S.E. (2004) Familial hypercholesterolemia and coronary heart disease: a HuGE association review. *American Journal of Epidemiology* 160, 421–429.

Austin, M.A., Hair, M.S. and Fullerton, S.M. (2012) Research guidelines in the era of large-scale collaborations: an analysis of genome-wide association study consortia. *American Journal of Epidemiology* 175, 962–969.

Bamshad, M.J., Ng, S.B., Bigham, A.W., Tabor, H.K., Emond, M.J., Nickerson, D.A. and Shendure J. (2011) Exome sequencing as a tool for Mendelian disease gene discovery. *Nature Reviews Genetics* 12, 745–755.

Behrman, R., Benner, J.S., Brown, J.S., McClellan, M., Woodcock, J. and Platt, R. (2011) Developing the sentinel system – a national resource for evidence development. *New England Journal of Medicine* 364, 498–499.

Bertina, R.M., Koeleman, B.P., Koster, T., Rosendaal, F.R., Dirven, R.J., de Ronde, H., *et al.* (1994) Mutation in blood coagulation factor V associated with resistance to activated protein C. *Nature* 369, 64–67.

Browning, S.R. (2008) Missing data imputation and haplotype phase inference for genome-wide association studies. *Human Genetics* 124, 439–450.

Cirulli, E.T. and Goldstein, D.B. (2010) Uncovering the roles of rare variants in common disease through whole-genome sequencing. *Nature Reviews Genetics* 11, 415–425.

Cohen, J.C., Kiss, R.S., Pertsemlidis, A., Marcel, Y.L., McPherson, R. and Hobbs, H.H. (2004) Multiple rare alleles contribute to low plasma levels of HDL cholesterol. *Science* 305, 869–872.

Cohorts for Heart and Aging Research in Genetic Epidemiology (CHARGE) Consortium (2012) Available from: http://web.chargeconsortium.com/ (accessed November 26, 2012).

Costa, L.G. and Eaton, D.L. (2006) *Gene–Environment Interaction. Fundamentals of Ecogenetics.* John Wiley & Sons, Hoboken, New Jersey, p. 3.

de Bakker, P.I., Burtt, N.P., Graham, R.R., Guiducci, C., Yelenskiy, R., Drake J.A., *et al.* (2006) Transferability of tag SNPs in genetic association studies in multiple populations. *Nature Genetics* 38, 1298–1303.

Dupuis, J., Langenberg, C., Prokopenko, I., Saxena, R., Soranzo, N., Jackson, A.U., *et al.* for the MAGIC investigators (2010) Novel genetic loci implicated in fasting glucose homeostatis and their impact on type 2 diabetes risk. *Nature Genetics* 42, 105–116.

Ehret, G.B., Munroe, P.B., Rice, K.M., Bochud, M., Johnson, A.D., Chasman, D.I., *et al.* for The International Consortium for Blood Pressure Genome-Wide Association Studies (2011) Genetic variants in novel pathways influence blood pressure and cardiovascular disease risk. *Nature* 478, 103–109.

Emerging Risk Factors Collaboration, Kaptoge, S., Di Angelantonio, E., Lowe, G., Pepys, M.B., Thompson, S.G., Collins, R. and Danesh, J. (2010) C-reactive protein concentration and risk of coronary heart disease, stroke, and mortality: an individual participant meta-analysis. *Lancet* 375, 1321–1340.

Emond, M.J., Louie, T., Emerson, J., Zhao, W., Mathias, R.A., Knowles, M.R., *et al.* (2012) Exome sequencing of extreme phenotypes identifies *DCTN4* as a modifier of chronic *Pseudomonas aeruginosa* infection in cystic fibrosis. *Nature Genetics* 44, 886–889.

Fisher, R.A. (1918) The correlation between relatives on the supposition of Mendelian inheritance. *Transactions of the Royal Society of Edinburgh* 52, 399–433.

Galton, F. (1886) Hereditary stature. *Nature* 33, 295–298.

Gehring, N.H., Frede, U., Neu-Yilik, G., Hundsdoerfer, P., Vetter, B., Hentze, M.W. and Kulozik, A.E. (2001) Increased efficiency of mRNA 3' end formation: a new genetic mechanism contributing to hereditary thrombophilia. *Nature Genetics* 28, 289–392.

Gelehrter, T.D., Collins, F.S. and Ginsburg, D. (1998) *Principles of Medical Genetics*, 2nd edn. Williams & Wilkins, Baltimore, Maryland, p. 49.

Gibson G. (2010) Hints of hidden heritability in GWAS. *Nature Genetics* 42, 558–560.

Gudbjartsson, D.F., Walters, G.B., Thorleifsson, G., Stefansson, H., Halldorsson, B.V., Zusmanovich, P., *et al.* (2008) Many sequence variants affecting diversity of adult human height. *Nature Genetics* 40, 609–615.

Hindorff, L., Sethupathy, P., Junkins, H., Ramos, E.M., Mehta, J.P., Collins, F.S. and Manolio, T.A. (2009) Potential etiologic and functional implications of genome-wide association loci for human diseases and traits. *Proceedings of the National Academy of Sciences USA* 106, 9362–9367.

Kanetsky, P.A., Mitra, N., Vardhanabhuti, S., Li, M., Vaughn, D.J., Letrero, R., *et al.* (2009) Common variation in *KITLG* and at 5q31.3 predisposes to testicular germ cell cancer. *Nature Genetics* 41, 811–815.

Kiezun, A., Garilmella, K., Do, R., Stitziel, N.O., Neale, B.M., McLaren, P.J., *et al.* (2012) Exome sequencing and the genetic basis of complex traits. *Nature Genetics* 44, 623–629.

Koepsell, T.D. and Weiss, N.S. (2003) Inferring a causal relation between exposure and disease. In: *Epidemiologic Methods. Studying the Occurrence of Illness*. Oxford University Press, New York, pp. 179–195.

Lander, E.S. (2012) Initial impact of the sequencing of the human genome. *Nature* 470, 187–197.

Lango Allen, H., Estrada, K., Lettre, G., Berndt, S., Weedon, M.N., Rivadeneira, F., *et al.* (2010) Hundreds of variants clustered in genomic loci and biological pathways affect human height. *Nature* 467, 832–838.

Lettre, G., Jackson, A.U., Gieger, C., Schumacher, F.R., Berndt, S.I., Sanna, S., *et al.* (2008) Identification of ten loci associated with height highlights new biological pathways in human growth. *Nature Genetics* 40, 584–591.

Levy, D., Ehret, G.B., Rice, K., Verwoert, G.C., Launer, L.J., Dehghan, A., *et al.* (2009) Association of common genetic variants with blood pressure and hypertension: a genome-wide association study of six population-based cohort studies, replication, and meta-analysis. *Nature Genetics* 41, 677–687.

Li, B. and Leal, S.M. (2008) Methods for detecting associations with rare variants for common diseases: application to the analysis of sequence data. *American Journal of Human Genetics* 83, 311–321.

Madsen, B.E. and Browning, S.R. (2009) A groupwise association test for rare mutations using a weighted sum statistic. *PLoS Genetics* 5, e1000384.

Manolio, T.A. (2010) Genomewide association studies and assessment of the risk of disease. *New England Journal of Medicine* 363, 166–176.

Manolio, T.A., Collins, F.S., Cox, N.J., Goldstein, D.B., Hindorff, L.A., Hunter, D.A., *et al.* (2009) Finding the missing heritability of complex diseases. *Nature* 461, 747–753.

McCarthy, M.I., Abecasis, G.R., Cardon, L.R., Goldstein, D.B., Little, J., Ioannidis, J.P.A. and Hirschhorn, J.N. (2008) Genome-wide association studies for complex traits: consensus, uncertainty and challenges. *Nature Reviews Genetics* 9, 356–369.

McClellan, J. and King, M.C. (2010) Genetic heterogeneity in human disease. *Cell* 141, 210–217.

Nature Encode Explorer (2012) Available from: www.nature.com/encode (accessed November 26, 2012).

Neale, B.M., Rivas, M.A., Voight, B.F., Altshuler, D., Devlin, B., Orho-Melander, M., *et al.* (2011) Testing for an unusual distribution of rare variants. *PLoS Genetics* 7, e1001322.

Newton-Cheh, C., Johnson, T., Gateva, V., Tobin, M.D., Cochud, M., Coin, L., *et al.* (2009) Eight blood pressure loci identified by genome-wide association study of 34,433 people of European ancestry. *Nature Genetics* 41, 666–676.

Ng, S.B., Turner, E.H., Robertson, P.D., Flygare, S.D., Bigham, A.W., Lee, C., *et al.* (2009) Targeted capture and massively parallel sequencing of 12 human exomes. *Nature* 461, 272–276.

Ng, S.B., Buckingham, K.J., Lee, C., Bigham, A.W., Tabor, H.K., Dent, K.M., *et al.* (2010a) Exome sequencing identifies the cause of a Mendelian disorder. *Nature Genetics* 42, 30–35.

Ng, S.G., Nickerson, D.A., Bamshad, M.J. and Shendure, J. (2010b) Massively parallel sequencing and rare disease. *Human Molecular Genetics* 19, R119–R124.

NHLBI Grand Opportunity Exome Sequencing Project (ESP). Available from: https://esp.gs.washington.edu/drupal/ (accessed November 26, 2012).

Ott, J., Kamatani, Y. and Lathrop, M. (2011) Family-based designs for genome-wide association studies. *Nature Reviews Genetics* 12, 465–474.

Park, J.-H., Wacholder, S., Gail, M.H., Peters, U., Jacobs, K.B., Chanock, S.J. and Chatterjee, N. (2010) Estimation of effect size distribution from genome-wide association studies and implications for future discoveries. *Nature Genetics* 42, 570–575.

Pearson, K. and Lee, A. (1903) On the laws of inheritance in man. I. Inheritance of physical characters. *Biometrika* 2, 357–462.

Pearson, T.A. and Manolio, T.A. (2008) How to interpret a genome-wide association study. *JAMA* 299, 1335–1344.

Poort, S.R., Rosendaal, F.R., Reitsma, P.H. and Bertina, R.M. (1996) A common genetic variation in the 3'-untranslated region of the prothrombin gene is associated with elevated plasma prothrombin levels and an increase in venous thrombosis. *Blood* 88, 3698–3703.

Pritchard, J.K. and Cox, N.J. (2002) The allelic architecture of human disease genes: common disease – common variant ... or not? *Human Molecular Genetics* 11, 2417–2423.

Psaty, B.M., O'Donnell, C.J., Gudnason, V., Lunetta, K.L., Folsom, A.R., Rotter, J.I., *et al.*, on Behalf of the CHARGE Consortium (2009) Cohorts for heart and aging research in genomic epidemiology (CHARGE): design of prospective meta-analyses of genome-wide association studies. *Circulation Cardiovascular Genetics* 2, 73–80.

Ridker, P.M., Hennekens, C.H., Lindpaintner, K., Eisenberg, P.R. and Miletich, J.P. (1995) Mutation in the gene coding for coagulation factor V and the risk of myocardial infarction, stroke, and venous thrombosis in apparently healthy men. *New England Journal of Medicine* 332, 912–917.

Risch, N. and Merikangas, K. (1996) The future of genetic studies of complex human diseases. *Science* 273, 1516–1517.

Rosendaal, F.R., Siscovick, D.S., Schwartz, S.M., Psaty, B.M., Raghunathan, T.E. and Vos, H.L. (1997) A common prothrombin variant (20210 G to A) increases the risk of myocardial infarction in young women. *Blood* 90, 1747–1750.

Sauna, Z.E. and Kimchi-Sarfaty, C. (2011) Understanding the contribution of synonymous mutations to human disease. *Nature Reviews Genetics* 12, 683–691.

Saxena, R., Hivert, M.F., Langenberg, C., Tanaka, T., Pankow, J.S., Vollenweider, P., *et al.* for the MAGIC investigators (2010) Genetic variation in gastric inhibitory polypeptide receptor (GIPR) impacts the glucose and insulin responses to an oral glucose challenge. *Nature Genetics* 42, 142–148.

Schaid, D.J. and Jacobsen, S.J. (1999) Biased tests of association: comparisons of allele frequencies when departing from Hardy–Weinberg proportion. *American Journal of Epidemiology* 149, 706–711.

Silventoinen, K. (2003) Determinants of variation in adult body height. *Journal of Biosocial Science* 35, 263–285.

Tabor, H.K., Risch, N.J. and Myers, R.M. (2002) Candidate-gene approaches for studying complex genetic traits: practical considerations. *Nature Review Genetics* 3, 391–397.

Tennessen, J.A., Bigham, A.W., O'Connor, T.D., Fu, W., Kenney, E.E., Simon, G., *et al.* (2012) Evolution and functional impact of rare coding variation from deep sequencing of human exomes. *Science* 337, 64–69.

Visscher, P.M. (2008) Sizing up human height variation. *Nature Genetics* 40, 489–490.

Visscher, P.M., Medland, S.E., Ferreira, M.A.R., Morley, K.I., Zhu, G., Cornes, B.K., *et al.* (2006) Assumption-free estimation of heritability from genome-wide identity-by-descent sharing between full siblings. *PLoS Genetics* 2, e41.

Visscher, P.M., Brown, M.A., McCarthy, M.I. and Yang, J. (2012) Five years of GWAS discovery. *American Journal of Human Genetics* 90, 7–24.

Wacholder, S., Chanock, S., Garcia-Closas, M., El Ghormli, L. and Rothman N. (2004) Assessing the probability that a positive report is false: an approach for molecular epidemiology studies. *Journal of the National Cancer Institute* 96, 434–442.

Wakefield, J. (2007) A Bayesian measure of the probability of false discovery in genetic epidemiology studies. *American Journal of Human Genetics* 81, 208–227.

Wang, S.S., Beaty, T.H. and Khoury, M.J. (2010) Genetic epidemiology. In: Speicher, M.R., Antonarakis, S.E., Motulsky, A.G., Vogel, F. and Motulsky, A.G. (eds) *Vogel and Motulsky's Human Genetics. Problems and Approaches*, 4th edn. Springer-Verlag, Berlin, pp. 617–634.

Weedon, M.N., Lango, H., Lindgren, C.M., Wallace, C., Evans, D.M., Mangino, M., *et al.* (2008) Genome-wide association analysis identifies 20 loci that influence adult height. *Nature Genetics* 40, 575–583.

Wolpin, B.M., Chan, A.T., Hartge, P., Chanock, S.J., Kraft, P., Hunter, D.J., *et al.* (2009) ABO blood group and the risk of pancreatic cancer. *Journal of the National Cancer Institute* 101, 424–431.

Xu, J., Turner, A., Little, J., Bleecker, E.R. and Meyers D.A. (2002) Positive results in association studies are associated with departure from Hardy–Weinberg equilibrium: hint for genotyping error? *Human Genetics* 111, 573–574.

Yang, J., Benyamin, B., McEvory, B.P., Gordon, S., Henders, A.K., Nyholt, D.R., *et al.* (2010) Common SNPs explain a large proportion of heritability for human height. *Nature Genetics* 42, 565–569.

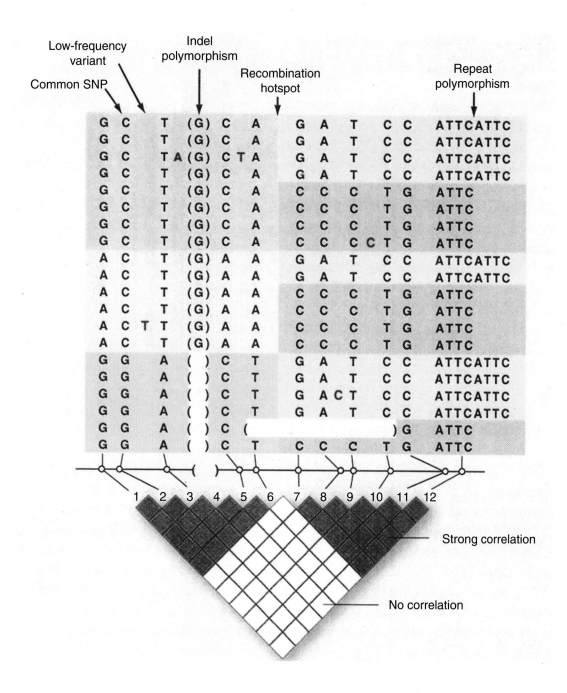

**Plate 1.** Illustration of types of genetic variants and markers in the human genome. (Reprinted with permission from Altshuler *et al.*, 2008.)

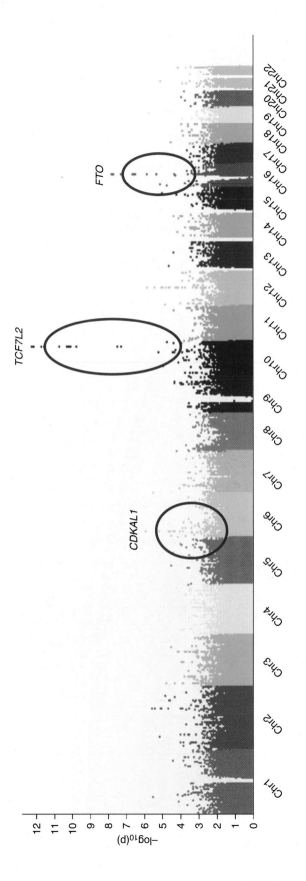

**Plate 2.** Manhattan plot from the Wellcome Trust Case Control Consortium GWAS of type 2 diabetes. The *x* axis represents chromosomal locations and the *y* axis shows *p*-values on a negative logarithmic scale. (Reprinted with permission from McCarthy *et al.*, 2008.)

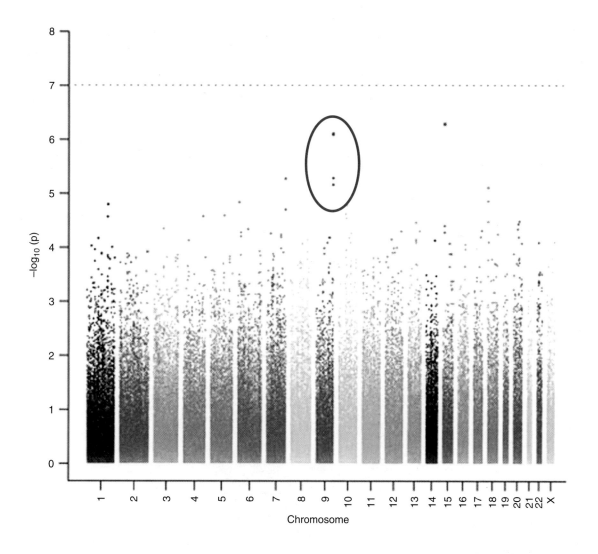

**Plate 3.** Manhattan plot for the genome-wide association study of pancreatic cancer for 12 cohort studies and one case–control study. (Reprinted with permission from Amundadottir *et al.*, 2009.)

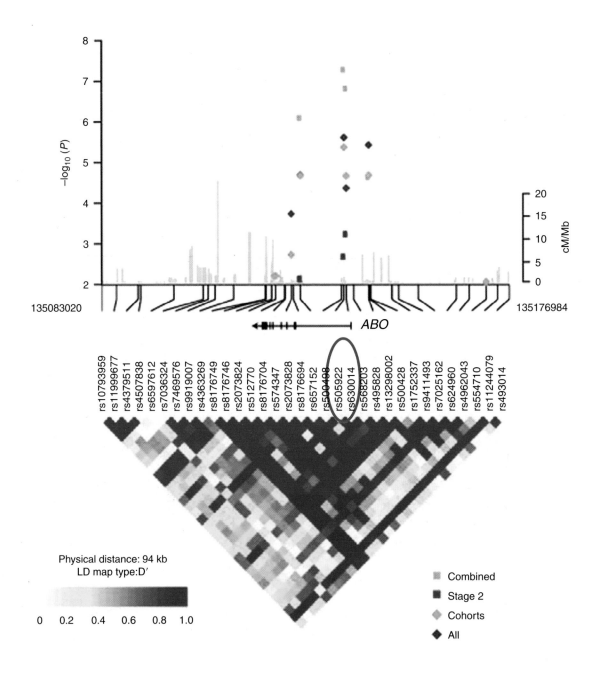

**Plate 4.** Association of SNPs in the region of the *ABO* gene on chromosome 9 with pancreatic cancer, estimated recombination rates, and linkage disequilibrium. (Reprinted with permission from Amundadottir *et al.*, 2009.)

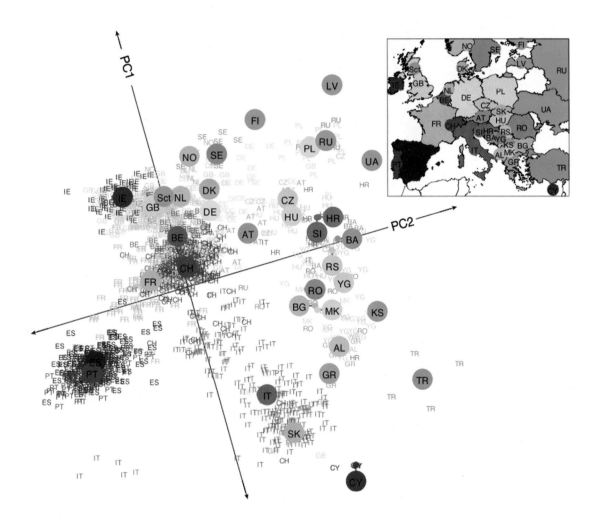

**Plate 5.** Population structure within Europe. A statistical summary of genetic data from 1387 Europeans based on principal component axis one (PC1) and axis two (PC2). Small colored labels represent individuals and large colored points represent median PC1 and PC2 values for each country. The inset map provides a key to the labels. The PC axes are rotated to emphasize the similarity to the geographic map of Europe. AL, Albania; AT, Austria; BA, Bosnia-Herzegovina; BE, Belgium; BG, Bulgaria; CH, Switzerland; CY, Cyprus; CZ, Czech Republic; DE, Germany; DK, Denmark; ES, Spain; FI, Finland; FR, France; GB, United Kingdom; GR, Greece; HR, Croatia; HU, Hungary; IE, Ireland; IT, Italy; KS, Kosovo; LV, Latvia; MK, Macedonia; NO, Norway; NL, Netherlands; PL, Poland; PT, Portugal; RO, Romania; RS, Serbia and Montenegro; RU, Russia; Sct, Scotland; SE, Sweden; SI, Slovenia; SK, Slovakia; TR, Turkey; UA, Ukraine; YG, Yugoslavia. (Reprinted with permission from Novembre *et al.*, 2008.)

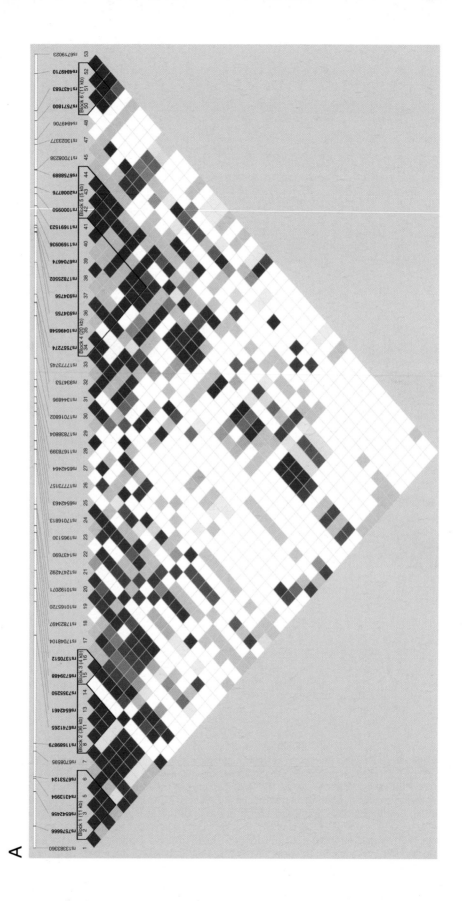

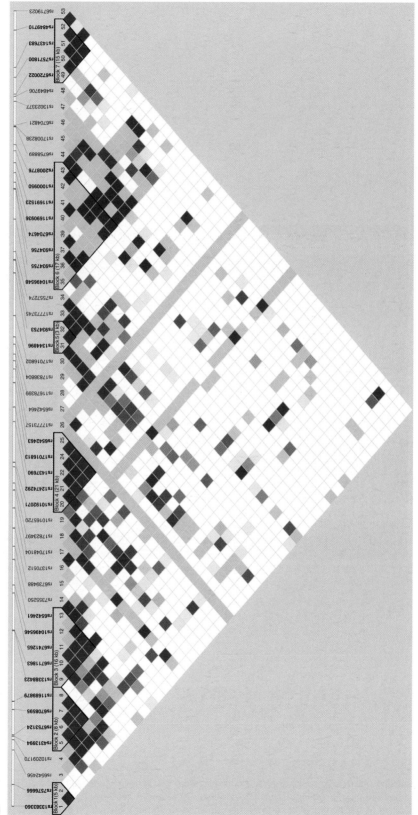

**Plate 6.** Linkage disequilibrium (LD) plots for the HapMap CEU (A) and YRI (B) with the Haploview software for a 200 kb region on chromosome 2. LD is based on the measures of D' and LOD (bright red, D' = 1 and LOD ≥ 2; shades of pink/red, D' < 1 and LOD ≥ 2; white, D' < 1 and LOD < 2; blue, D' = 1 and LOD < 2).

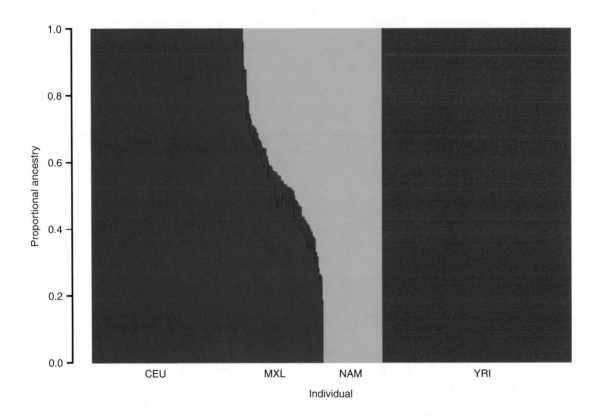

**Plate 7.** Supervised individual ancestry analysis for the HapMap MXL sample where the HapMap CEU and YRI samples were included as fixed groups in the analysis for European (blue) and African (red) ancestry, respectively, and HGDP NAM were included as a fixed group for Native American ancestry (green). Each individual is represented by a vertical bar with proportional ancestry contributions color coded on the *y* axis.

# 6  Population Stratification in Genetic Association Studies

BARBARA MCKNIGHT, PH.D.

*Department of Biostatistics, University of Washington, Seattle, Washington*

## Synopsis

- In evaluating evidence from genome-wide association studies (GWAS) of unrelated subjects, analysts must take care to avoid confounding by differences in allelic frequency that are associated with the trait for reasons other than a direct genetic influence, termed population stratification.
- "Global" population stratification occurs when subgroups of the study population have a specific ancestry that is associated both with allele frequencies at loci throughout the genome and also with the trait.
- "Local" structure occurs in recently admixed populations where alleles have different frequencies in the different ancestral populations, or where they have been subject to recent natural selection in the admixed population, resulting in confounding at one or more moderately large haplotypes.
- Several statistical procedures can detect and control population stratification, both global and local.
- The analysis of GWAS data should always include evaluation of the possible role of population stratification confounding, and when it is present, should always use available statistical methods to control it.

## 6.1  General Concepts

### 6.1.1  Rationale for GWAS

The motivation for GWAS is the idea that common genetic variation is associated with disease phenotypes of interest in the population. Common causal variants probably arose many generations ago, and were not so strongly associated with reproductive fitness that they have been eliminated by natural selection. The left side of Fig. 6.1 depicts how this might have happened. If in the past a mutation (black dots) created a causal variant, after many generations and meioses, many copies of this variant exist in the population, and multiple recombination events have left only those genetic loci in close proximity to it still associated. The causal variant and nearby alleles from the haplotype where the mutation originally occurred have been inherited together through the generations, and particular alleles at nearby genetic markers (denoted b for one marker in Fig. 6.1) are still associated with the causal variant in the population. Variation at single nucleotide polymorphisms (SNPs) near the causal

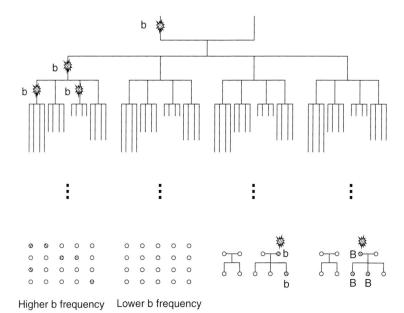

Higher b frequency    Lower b frequency

**Fig. 6.1.** Comparison of the inheritance of old, common trait-influencing mutations (black dots) and nearby markers with the inheritance of newer, rarer trait-influencing mutations (black stripes) and less nearby markers within families. Alleles at the markers near to old, common mutations are now associated with the trait population-wide; alleles at the markers near the newer, rarer mutations may now be associated with the trait only within families.

locus is now associated with the trait, and population-wide association of SNP genotype with trait can identify regions where a causal locus is likely to reside (Risch and Merikangas, 1996).

This population history contrasts with a history of multiple, more recent, and still very rare mutations that can be detected by genetic linkage analysis in families. Because fewer generations have passed and fewer meioses have occurred, marker genotypes over a much larger genetic region are correlated with the causal variant and trait within families, but from family to family the marker genotype that is associated with the trait may differ. This population history is depicted in the right half of Fig. 6.1, where, depending on the family, it is either the allele b or the allele B that is associated with the causal mutation (black stripes) and the trait. A GWAS of unrelated individuals has little power to detect this locus without a huge sample size and genetic sequencing data, or a SNP that is the actual causal variant. This is because no particular marker allele is associated population-wide with the causal variant, and the variant may be very rare.

### 6.1.2  Population stratification confounding

Epidemiologists are well aware of the problem of confounding in observational data. Studying the causal association between risk factors and disease, an attribute that increases the likelihood of exposure to the risk factor and also increases the risk of disease,

B. McKnight

will create a spurious association between the risk factor and the disease. This spurious association can be removed by considering the association of risk factor and disease among subjects with like values of the attribute, using statistical regression methods for adjustment, or by standardizing so that the analysis compares exposed and unexposed populations with the same distribution of the attribute (Koepsell and Weiss, 2003).

Although environmental exposures are not thought to influence genotype, confounding can still occur in GWAS; the reason is usually differences in ethnicity. Distinct ethnic groups have distinct allele frequencies at many loci, and in an ethnically diverse population, ethnicity-related differences in genotype may appear to be associated with a trait because genotype at an entirely different locus, also correlated with ethnicity, influences the trait. Distinct ethnic groups also often share distinct dietary habits and other lifestyle characteristics, and these differences may cause the trait to be associated with ethnic group. When this happens, any genotype that is more frequent in an ethnic group with higher or lower values of the trait will appear to be associated with the trait in an ethnically mixed population. This population structure is referred to as "population stratification": the population under study is composed of strata formed by ethnic groups that have different trait distributions and different genotype distributions.

Figure 6.2 illustrates population stratification confounding for a hypothetical case–control study. Horizontal lines in each group show the genotype of an individual in that group: white denotes the presence of a minor allele. In Fig. 6.2a, the minor allele appears to be associated with case status. However, when we reorder

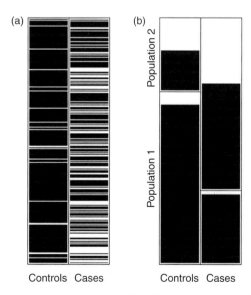

**Fig. 6.2.** Graphical depiction of population stratification confounding. Within case and control groups, white horizontal lines indicate a subject with at least one variant allele at the marker locus and black horizontal lines indicate a subject with two wild-type alleles at the locus.
(a) The case and control subjects are not sorted by subpopulation or marker genotype.
(b) The case and control subjects are sorted by both subpopulation and genotype.

the horizontal lines, grouping them by subpopulation and genotype in Fig. 6.2b, we see that there is little or no association between the presence of the minor allele and case status within each subpopulation.

Additional mechanisms can cause confounding in GWAS. If related individuals are contained in the sample, each family can act like a small ethnic group, with family-specific genotypes and lifestyle. When family membership is known, statistical methods for correlated data that use family information such as mixed models or generalized estimating equations should be used to analyze the data. However, sometimes closely related individuals are part of the sample but we do not know it; we call this "cryptic relatedness." Some of the diagnostic methods described in this chapter can detect confounding due to cryptic relatedness when it exists, but statistical methods to correct for it are specialized, and detailed descriptions of them appear elsewhere (Thornton and McPeek, 2007; Choi *et al.*, 2009; Kang *et al.*, 2010).

Age can also act as a confounder in GWAS, particularly in populations where, because of recent immigration patterns, different ages have different ethnic distributions. On any date where a trait is measured, the subjects' birth years may be associated not only with the trait value, but also with ethnicity and therefore genotype at many loci.

We encountered likely population stratification confounding in the analysis of data to be contributed to a GWAS of plasma phospholipid docosahexaenoic acid (DHA) in the Cardiovascular Health Study (CHS) (Lemaitre *et al.*, 2011). Circulating DHA levels are known to be related to fatty-fish consumption, and fatty-fish consumption may be associated with ethnicity. Without the diagnostic and corrective measures described in the next section, we might have reported many false associations. A more detailed description of our work is given in Box 6.1.

## 6.2 Detecting Population Stratification

When data on ethnicity or its correlates are available, GWAS association results can be adjusted for these variables using standard regression techniques to control confounding. The problem for GWAS is that detailed ethnicity data are often not available, and we must use other means to determine if population stratification is inflating the observed association between genetic variants and a trait.

The quantile–quantile or QQ plot is a useful diagnostic for detecting population stratification. This plot compares the observed distribution of p-values to what would be expected if the global null hypothesis of no genetic association with the trait were true. When there are no true genetic associations with the trait, and the number of subjects and minor allele frequency are both large enough that the approximate test-statistic distributions we use are adequate, we expect each p-value to have a Uniform[0,1] distribution. Although the p-values are not independent of each other because of the linkage disequilibrium (LD) between nearby SNPs, it has still been useful to treat the p-values as if they behaved like an independent sample of size n from a Uniform[0,1] distribution. Under this approximation, we can compare our smallest p-value to the expected value, $1/(n + 1)$, of the smallest value from a sample of n independent variables from a Uniform[0,1] distribution, compare the second smallest p-value to the expected value, $2/(n + 1)$, of the second smallest value in a sample

B. McKnight

of n from a Uniform[0,1] distribution, and so on. In practice, we do this graphically, and to highlight the distribution of the very smallest p-values, we plot the observed versus expected values of $-\log_{10}(p)$ rather than of p. The $-\log_{10}$ transformation has two virtues: it consolidates the uninteresting, large p-values into the bottom left corner of the plot, and the value of $-\log_{10}(p)$ readily shows the order of magnitude of the p-value; when $p = 0.0001 = 10^{-4}$, for example, $-\log_{10}(p) = 4$.

Figure 6.3 shows a QQ plot of observed and expected $-\log_{10}(p\text{-values})$ for 2.5 million hypothetical p-values drawn from a Uniform[0,1] distribution. The diagonal line shows what would be expected if the observed value always exactly equaled the expected, and the area between the dotted curves gives pointwise 95% prediction intervals. As expected, the observed values are very similar to the expected, and no point deviates from what would be expected based on the uniform distribution of the data.

For traits governed partially by genetic variation at one or more loci, we do expect some deviation from this expectation. SNPs in LD with any causal locus will be associated with the trait, and tests of association for these SNPs will yield lower than expected p-values. However, the associated SNPs will be few in number compared to the large number (often ~2.5 million) of association tests we perform, so the vast majority of p-values will follow the expected null hypothesis distribution. Figure 6.4 shows a QQ plot exhibiting this pattern: the smallest P-values deviate from the expected distribution, but the bulk of the p-values follow it.

When there is population stratification confounding, the points on the QQ plot take a different, characteristic shape. The ethnic subpopulation with differing values of the trait will usually have a different distribution of genotypes throughout the genome, so a large number of tests will be subject to confounding bias, their test-statistic values will be inflated, and their p-values will be artificially more significant than expected. This means the entire distribution of p-values will be lower than expected. Figure 6.5 shows the characteristic QQ plot, with $-\log_{10}(p)$ too high throughout the distribution: this pattern indicates a problem with cryptic relatedness or population stratification confounding.

There is one practical issue associated with the QQ plot diagnostic for GWAS: plotting 2.5 million points on a plot can take non-negligible computer time. Two useful

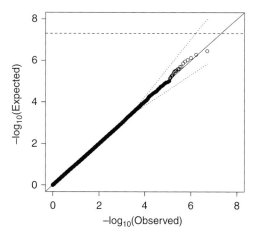

**Fig. 6.3.** Example expected pattern for a quantile–quantile plot of 2.5 million observed versus expected $-\log_{10}(p\text{-values})$ if there is no population stratification or cryptic relatedness and no evidence of genetic association with the trait. Points should fall on or near the diagonal line, within the boundaries indicated with the short dashed lines. The longer, horizontal dashed line indicates a common boundary above which $-\log_{10}$ p-values are declared genome-wide significant.

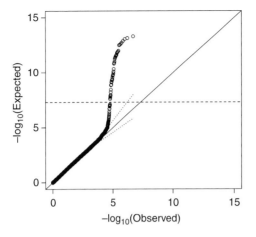

**Fig. 6.4.** Example expected pattern for a quantile–quantile plot of 2.5 million observed versus expected $-\log_{10}$(p-values) if there is no population stratification or cryptic relatedness but there is evidence of genetic association with the trait at one or more loci. For SNPs at or near associated loci, the largest observed $-\log_{10}$(p-values) are larger than expected under the global null hypothesis.

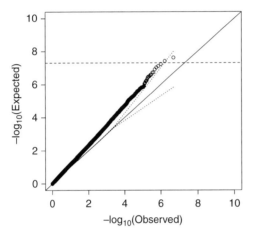

**Fig. 6.5.** Example expected pattern for a quantile–quantile plot of 2.5 million observed versus expected $-\log_{10}$(p-values) if there is population stratification or cryptic relatedness but no evidence of genetic association with the trait. For many SNPs throughout the genome, the observed $-\log_{10}$(p-values) are larger than expected under the global null hypothesis.

ways to reduce the time required are hexagonal bin plotting (Carr *et al.*, 1987) and plotting only the points associated with p-values less than some threshold. Hexagonal bin plotting divides the plotting plane into small hexagons, and fills each hexagon with a symbol sized proportionally to the number of points that fall in the hexagon. Figure 6.6 is a hexagonal bin plot for the same p-values shown in Fig. 6.5; it was created with the R package Hexbin. The line clearly deviates from the expected slope of one. This is also shown in Fig. 6.7, where only points for which the expected p-value is less than 0.001 are plotted. At 0.001, it is easy to see that the distribution has departed importantly from what would be expected if there were few genetic associations and no population stratification confounding, and only 0.1% of the original points are plotted. Figures 6.5, 6.6, and 6.7 all signal the presence of population stratification confounding or cryptic relatedness, and the need for one or more of the correction methods described in the next section.

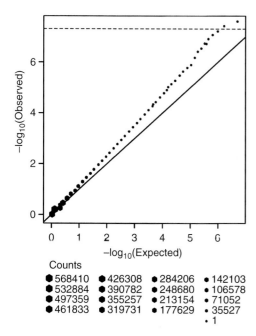

Counts
- ● 568410  ● 426308  ● 284206  • 142103
- ● 532884  ● 390782  ● 248680  • 106578
- ● 497359  ● 355257  ● 213154  • 71052
- ● 461833  ● 319731  • 177629  • 35527
- • 1

**Fig. 6.6.** Hexagonal bin plot of the observed versus expected $-\log_{10}$(p-value) data in Fig. 6.5. The plane is divided into invisible hexagons of the same size, and the size of the black fill within each hexagon is associated with the number of points falling in that hexagon.

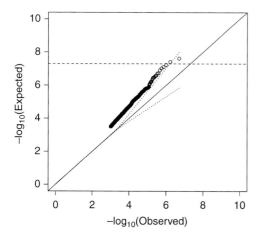

**Fig. 6.7.** Plot of the observed versus expected $-\log_{10}$(p-value) data in Fig. 6.5, but with only the points where $p < 10^{-3}$ plotted.

## 6.3 Statistical Methods to Adjust for Global Population Stratification Confounding

### 6.3.1 Genomic control

One of the first statistical methods suggested to correct for test-statistic inflation owing to population-stratification confounding and cryptic relatedness was genomic control (Devlin and Roeder, 1999). Originally envisaged for application in candidate gene studies where genotype data might also be available for unrelated markers, it is based on estimating the amount by which the distribution of test statistics for assumed-null markers is inflated, compared to what would be expected if there were no confounding, and correcting each test statistic for this inflation.

If confounding inflates test-statistic values for these assumed-null SNPs, the inflation probably affects the entire distribution of test statistics, and the median of the distribution will be larger than expected. Assuming that the squared, two-sided version of most test statistics used in GWAS will be compared to their large-sample approximate $\chi^2_1$ distribution, the genomic-control $\lambda$ is the ratio of the median of the observed null test-statistic values to the median of the $\chi^2_1$ distribution, 0.4549. The value of $\lambda$ will be greater than one when the test-statistic values are inflated by population-stratification confounding. The correction then consists of dividing all test statistics by $\lambda$ to correct for the observed amount of inflation, before computing p-values. When the signed, square-root version of the test statistic is used and compared to a standard normal distribution, the equivalent correction divides the test statistic by the square root of $\lambda$.

In GWAS, we have not usually identified a set of SNPs assumed to be unrelated to the trait. In almost all GWAS, we assume, however, that the number of loci truly related to the trait is relatively small, so that the vast majority of SNPs are not associated. The few SNPs that do show an association with the trait will have little effect on the median value of all the test statistics, so for GWAS it has become standard practice to base the calculation of $\lambda$ on the median of all the GWAS test statistics. When the p-values in Fig. 6.5 were subjected to genomic control, $\lambda$ was computed to be 1.200; Fig. 6.8 shows how the genomic-control-corrected QQ plot for the same tests removes the inflation. Before genomic control, the smallest p-value in the figure was $2.4 \times 10^{-8}$ and the tenth smallest was $2.6 \times 10^{-7}$; after correction these values were $3.5 \times 10^{-7}$ and $2.6 \times 10^{-6}$, respectively.

The genomic-control method has been studied in a number of settings (Marchini *et al.*, 2004; Price *et al.*, 2010; Bouaziz *et al.*, 2011; Wu *et al.*, 2011) and found to perform poorly when there is a large degree of population stratification confounding, or when the test-statistic inflation is due to cryptic relatedness rather than population stratification. In population-stratification settings most relevant for GWAS, where a large number of SNPs are used to estimate $\lambda$ and when there are large differences between subpopulations, the method can be very conservative, meaning it yields too many false-negative results (Marchini *et al.*, 2004; Bouaziz *et al.*, 2011; Wu *et al.*, 2011).

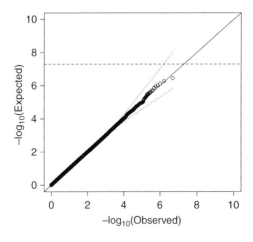

**Fig. 6.8.** Quantile–quantile plot of 2.5 million observed versus expected $-\log_{10}$ (p-values) for the same example data plotted in Figs 6.5–6.7, after correction by genomic control.

B. McKnight

When $\lambda < 1.05$, the genomic-control correction is usually considered adequate (Price *et al.*, 2010) but when the amount of inflation is greater than this, one or more of the adjustment methods in the following sections may be necessary.

### 6.3.2 Ethnicity adjustment

In the rare case where detailed, accurate data on ethnic origin are available, and little ethnic admixture is present, it is possible that the ethnicity data are adequate to control for population-stratification confounding bias. In principle, letting $f(Y)$ denote the general trait outcome parameter modeled (mean for linear regression, logit(p) for logistic regression, and log hazard – with a function of time for intercept – for Cox regression), when we let g denote the number of minor alleles at the SNP of interest, let X be a matrix of indicators for different ethnic groups, and let Z be a matrix of any other adjustment variables, the model:

$$f(Y) = \beta_0 + \beta_1 X + \beta_2 Z + \beta_3 g$$

could, in principle, provide inference about $\beta_3$ that controls for the confounding effect of ethnic group. In practice, however, it is unlikely that the investigator would be able to tell whether the ethnicity data available were detailed enough to accomplish this. We often perform a crude version of this type of ethnicity adjustment by restricting each single GWAS analysis to subjects of the same racial group.

### 6.3.3 Principal components adjustment

One very attractive approach that has proved useful in controlling population stratification bias is adjustment for principal components, also known as the EIGENSTRAT or EIGENSOFT method (EIGENSOFT; Price *et al.*, 2006). In this method, the first principal components of the GWAS SNPs are computed and included as independent variables in regression models relating SNP genotype to trait.

The first principal components are designed to summarize most of the variation in a large number of variables with many fewer variables. In general for any n variables $X_1, \ldots X_n$, the first principal component is the linear combination $a_1 X_1 + \ldots + a_n X_n$ with the largest observed variance. The second principal component is the linear combination $a'_1 X_1 + \ldots + a'_n X_n$, with largest observed variance among linear combinations uncorrelated with the first principal component, and so on. Figure 6.9 shows how the first principal component of a set of two continuous variables finds the direction with the most variation. The values of the principal components are the coordinates of each point on the appropriate principal component axes, PC1 and PC2 in Fig. 6.9. When $X_1, \ldots X_n$ count alleles at SNPs, Price *et al.* (2006) have called these coordinates "ancestries."

Letting X be a matrix of the first n SNP principal components, we will use the same notation for g = SNP, Z = adjustment variables, and Y = outcome as in Section 6.3.2. We can fit the model:

$$f(Y) = \beta_0 + \beta_1 X + \beta_2 Z + \beta_3 g \tag{6.1}$$

for each SNP g separately to adjust for ethnicity. This analysis can be performed in special-purpose software (EIGENSOFT) or in any standard statistical package. Price and colleagues (2006) recommend using the first ten principal components.

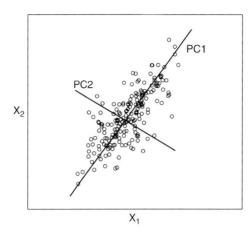

$X_2$

$X_1$

**Fig. 6.9.** Scatterplot of hypothetical data on two continuous variables $x_1$ and $x_2$, with lines depicting the two principal component axes superimposed.

In GWAS data, it is often true that even fewer principal components account for a large part of the ethnic variation in SNP genotypes, and adjustment for these in a regression model adequately controls confounding by population structure. Indeed, a recent application of principal components to genetic data by Novembre *et al.* (2008) showed that, among Europeans for whom all four grandparents originated in the same country, the first two principal components computed from approximately 200,000 nearly uncorrelated SNPs could map their country of origin fairly accurately in the plane; see Plate 5. Examining QQ plots after performing a principal-components-adjusted analysis can verify that enough principal components have been included to control the important genetic similarities.

Simulation studies of association testing under models of admixture report that adjustment for principal components usually works well to control population stratification confounding (Price *et al.*, 2010; Bouaziz *et al.*, 2011; Wu *et al.*, 2011), though when the phenotype values vary across subpopulations but the SNP does not, adjustment for principal components can reduce power (Peloso and Lunetta, 2011).

### 6.3.4 Estimated ancestry adjustment

Another way to account for ancestry is to estimate the proportion of a subject's alleles arising from each of several ancestral populations and to adjust for these estimated proportions in the model for SNP–phenotype association by replacing the principal components in X with them in Eqn 6.1. An early method for imputing ancestries was implemented in publically available software (STRUCTURE), which estimates the proportion of alleles arising from each of K putative ancestral populations under a Bayesian model using Markov chain Monte Carlo methods (Pritchard *et al.* 2000). Under the assumption that any Hardy–Weinberg disequilibrium or LD between distant loci is due to population structure, the procedure provides posterior modes to estimate the proportions $(p_1, p_2, \ldots p_K)$ of each individual's genome derived from each of K ancestral populations. This method was soon extended (Falush *et al.*, 2003) to accommodate linked markers. The STRUCTURE algorithm is time-consuming, and not practical for most large-scale GWAS, though with enrichment from different HAPMAP samples, it has been used to restrict subjects to those with common ancestry (Sladek *et al.*, 2007; Thomas *et al.*, 2009). Tang *et al.* (2005) developed a more computationally efficient

B. McKnight

maximum-likelihood approach to estimating $(p_1, p_2, \ldots p_K)$ that has been used to study how genetic similarity is associated with what is known about the world history of migration patterns (Li *et al.*, 2008); this has been implemented in publically available software (FRAPPE) and the algorithm is significantly faster than STRUCTURE. More recently, an even faster and very accurate algorithm has been developed (Alexander *et al.*, 2009; Alexander and Lange, 2011); it is also publicly available (ADMIXTURE).

### 6.3.5  Estimated correlation methods

Motivated primarily by controlling confounding due to cryptic relatedness, several recently proposed methods incorporate information about genetic correlation between individuals coming directly from study SNP data. The EMMAX method estimates the variance–covariance matrix for the phenotype by first estimating a kinship matrix from the SNP data, transforming it into the implied phenotype correlation matrix based on an underlying mixed model, and incorporating this into a variance components analysis (EMMAX; Kang *et al.*, 2010). The procedure then fits a general linear model for SNP–phenotype association by generalized least squares using this estimated covariance matrix as known. The authors show that this approach controls confounding better than adjusting for the first 100 principal components in the Wellcome Trust Case Control Consortium (Burton *et al.*, 2007) and Northern Finland Birth Cohort (Sabatti, 2008) data. The method has been used to control possible population structure confounding in several recent GWAS (Kullo *et al.*, 2011; Winkelmann *et al.*, 2011).

An alternative method, implemented in the ROADTRIPS software, reverses the role of outcome and independent variable in the usual regression model formulation (ROADTRIPS; Thornton and McPeek, 2010). Treating the multivariate SNP data as the outcome and the phenotype data as the independent variable, it estimates a correlation matrix for study subjects' SNP data, and then estimates the standard error for a possibly

---

**Box 6.1. Application: GWAS of DHA in the Cardiovascular Health Study (CHS)**

We recently reported associations of several genetic loci with long-chain n-3 polyunsaturated fatty acids in a meta-analysis of GWAS from a number of studies of subjects of European descent, including the CHS (Lemaitre *et al.*, 2011). Early GWAS analyses for several phenotypes in CHS using QQ plots had indicated no evidence of population stratification in this cohort after adjustment was made for age, sex, and each of the four US study sites, so we were not in the habit of adjusting for principal components. As part of our usual model checking in CHS, however, we examined QQ plots, and for the phenotype DHA we were surprised to find strong evidence of confounding (Fig. 6.10). Because levels of DHA are associated with levels of fatty-fish consumption, and because fatty-fish consumption might be associated with ethnicity, we suspected that population stratification could be the explanation. Figure 6.11 shows the QQ plot for the same associations, after adjustment for age, sex, study site and the first 30 principal components based on CHS GWAS data. The genomic-control $\lambda$ for Fig. 6.11 is 1.04. After making the genomic-control correction on these principal-component-adjusted tests, Fig. 6.12 shows the QQ plot based on p-values that were included in the meta-analysis.

*Continued*

---

Population Stratification in Association Studies

**Box 6.1.** Continued.

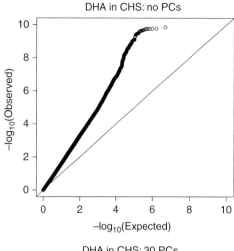

DHA in CHS: no PCs

**Fig. 6.10.** Quantile–quantile plot of observed versus expected $-\log_{10}$ (p-values) from the CHS GWAS of DHA with no principal components (PCs). Tests were adjusted for age, sex, and CHS site only.

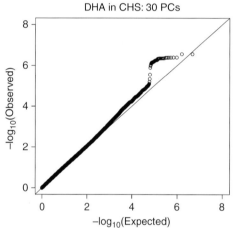

DHA in CHS: 30 PCs

**Fig. 6.11.** Quantile–quantile plot of observed versus expected $-\log_{10}$ (p-values) from the same CHS GWAS as in Fig. 6.10. Tests were adjusted for age, sex, CHS site, and the first 30 principal components.

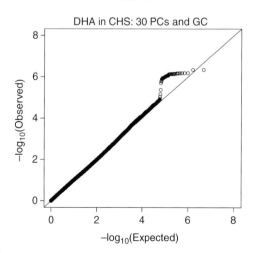

DHA in CHS: 30 PCs and GC

**Fig. 6.12.** Quantile–quantile plot of observed versus expected $-\log_{10}$ (p-values) from the same tests shown in Fig. 6.11, after adjustment using genomic control (GC).

B. McKnight

weighted regression score incorporating information about subject genetic correlations from this estimate. Recent simulation studies (Price *et al.*, 2010; Wu *et al.*, 2011) have shown that, although both of these methods do a good job of controlling confounding owing to cryptic relatedness, when population-stratification confounding is strong they can fail to control it in settings where adjusting for principal components works well.

## 6.4 Statistical Methods to Adjust for Local Population Stratification Confounding

When the population being studied in a GWAS has undergone recent admixture, the methods outlined in Section 6.3 may not be enough to avoid confounding bias. Local variation in ancestry can cause confounding of association results that may be difficult or impossible to detect and correct using the methods for global population structure confounding. This section explains how local population structure can come about, how it can affect GWAS, and how some recent proposals correct for possible bias.

### 6.4.1 Mixing of populations and local population structure

When two genetically distinct populations first mix, one copy of each chromosome in their offspring will derive from one of the two ancestral populations. In subsequent generations, recombination will mix genetic information from each of the ancestral populations on the same chromosome, and after several generations an individual chromosome may carry several long haplotypes, each haplotype deriving wholly from one of the two ancestral populations. After several generations in admixed populations, this process creates a population structure that is specific to moderately large regions of a single chromosome (local), but not detectable by methods assuming similar structure across the entire genome (global). Bonnen *et al.* (2009) estimated haplotype lengths in an admixed population in Micronesia that were consistent with the theoretically derived expected length of (100 centiMorgans)/k, where k is the number of meioses that have occurred since admixture (k = 1 for grandchildren of mixing members of the ancestral populations).

When the trait-influencing gene and a marker have different frequencies in the two ancestral populations, this structure in the admixed population could create a spurious association between traits influenced by genetic loci in one part of the haplotype and markers, fairly distant, that are still located in the same haplotype. Only adjustment for the ancestral source of the local genome could control for this.

In fact, even when the marker has the same frequency and the trait has the same distribution in the two ancestral populations, selection in the admixed population could create local population stratification confounding. Admixed populations sometimes form when one or more populations migrate to a new geographic region and mix with each other or with the indigenous population. Genes that have little influence on reproductive fitness in the old environment may become advantageous or deleterious in the new, and haplotypes derived from a migrating population and carrying advantageous variants will become more frequent in the admixed population in the new environment. Evidence for natural selection in admixed populations has been accumulating recently. For example, Tang *et al.* (2007) found evidence of recent natural selection in three genetic locations, including the human leukocyte antigen (HLA) region, among admixed Puerto Ricans.

Figure 6.13 shows how this could happen, and how it might affect inference about marker-trait association. At the Aa locus, allele a influences the trait. Genotype at the Bb locus is not associated with genotype at the Aa locus in either ancestral population and is distant from it, but still on the same haplotype for most members of the recently admixed population. The trait distribution and allele frequencies at the Aa and Bb loci are the same in both ancestral populations. But ab haplotypes in population 2 also carry the c allele at the Cc locus, and though it does not influence reproductive fitness in the old environment, it confers selective advantage in the new. This means that, after a few generations in the admixed population, the abc haplotype is more frequent than it is in either ancestral population, and the b allele at the Bb marker appears associated with the trait, even though it is quite distant from the causal Aa locus. In this example, local population stratification due to selection could exist even though the marker and trait gene were independent of each other and had the same distribution in both ancestral populations. In fact, the Aa and Bb loci would not even have to be on the same haplotype, or even on the same chromosome, for this bias to occur if the two haplotypes containing them were subject to similar selective pressures in the new environment.

### 6.4.2 Lactase persistence gene

Other mechanisms involving selection can also create local population-stratification confounding. Local geographic variation in environment that may be associated by chance with migration patterns and the trait-influencing genes could also create a spurious association between genes if the selection pressures were stronger in some locations than others. Campbell *et al.* (2005) found evidence that variation in the lactase persistence gene, probably conferring selective advantage in north-west but not south-east Europe, was associated with height in a population of mixed European descent. They found no association between this genotype and height in Poles or Scandinavians who were each more genetically similar to each other and were subject, within each country, to similar selective pressures.

After a few generations have passed in an admixed population, the population structure in the admixed population will be local only. Global diagnostics such as the QQ plot will fail to detect confounding resulting from local structure, and global

| | Population 1 | | | | Population 2 | | | |
|---|---|---|---|---|---|---|---|---|
| Trait: | A | A | a | a | A | A | a | a |
| Marker: | B | b | B | b | B | b | B | b |
| | C | C | C | C | C | C | C | c |
| Frequency: | $\frac{9}{20}$ | $\frac{9}{20}$ | $\frac{1}{20}$ | $\frac{1}{20}$ | $\frac{9}{20}$ | $\frac{9}{20}$ | $\frac{1}{20}$ | $\frac{1}{20}$ |

| | Admixed | | | | |
|---|---|---|---|---|---|
| Trait: | A | A | a | a | a |
| Marker: | B | b | B | b | b |
| Selective advantage: | C | C | C | C | c |
| Frequency: | $\frac{16}{40}$ | $\frac{16}{40}$ | $\frac{1}{40}$ | $\frac{1}{40}$ | $\frac{6}{40}$ |

**Fig. 6.13.** Haplotype frequencies for two ancestral populations and a population where these two have been admixed. Allele c at the Cc locus confers a selective advantage in the admixed population environment, making the abc haplotype more common there than would otherwise be expected.

correction measures including adjusting for global principal components or estimating the global proportion of genetic information from ancestral populations will fail to correct it (Campbell *et al.*, 2005). Association studies performed in recently admixed populations may need to account for local population structure to avoid confounding bias. The next section describes several recently proposed methods.

### 6.4.3 Controlling for local ancestry

Qin *et al.* (2010) described a local principal components method that was able to preserve the level of hypothesis tests better than global methods and that retained power in simulation studies when there was local population structure confounding. The method is based on dividing the genome into 4 Mb core intervals, and computing local principal components based on genetic information from the core interval and flanking intervals of up to 8 Mb on either side of the core; except near the telomeres and centromeres, the principal components are based on variation over a 20 Mb region. For each SNP within the core, the association test adjusts for the first ten of these local principal components. The authors note that it would be better to compute a separate set of principal components (from a 20 Mb surrounding window) for each SNP, but that this strategy is currently computationally prohibitive.

A simple method proposed recently (Wang *et al.*, 2011) estimates local ancestry for each SNP separately using recently developed algorithms for admixture mapping (HAPMIX; Pritchard *et al.*, 2009). The local ancestry estimate can then be incorporated as an adjustment variable in the regression model relating SNP to trait as described in Eqn 6.1 for principal components adjustment and global ancestry adjustment. Based on simulation studies, adjustment for estimated local ancestry appears to preserve the level of tests compared to global ancestry adjustments, and achieves good power. It has been used to control for local ancestry at top SNPs in a recent GWAS of African Americans (Reiner *et al.*, 2011).

## 6.5 Conclusion

GWAS of unrelated subjects can yield important information about the association between genetic loci and human traits. In evaluating the evidence for association between genetic loci and a trait, analysts must take care to avoid confounding by differences in allelic frequency that are associated with the trait for reasons other than a direct genetic influence. When subgroups of the study population have a specific ancestry that is associated both with many allele frequencies and also with the trait, this confounding can be present at loci throughout the genome (global population stratification). In recently admixed populations where alleles have different frequencies in the different ancestral populations, or where they have been subject to recent natural selection in the admixed population, confounding can also be present only in one or more moderately large haplotypes (local structure).

This chapter has described a number of statistical procedures that can detect and control population stratification, both global and local. The analysis of GWAS data should always include evaluation of the possible role of population stratification confounding, and, when it is present, should always use available statistical methods to control it.

## Acknowledgments

Preparation of this chapter was supported in part by grant DK089256 from the National Institute for Diabetes, Digestive and Kidney Diseases, and grants HL-085710 and HL-105756 from the National Heart, Lung, and Blood Institute.

CHS research was supported by NHLBI contracts N01-HC-85239, N01-HC-85079–N01-HC-85086, N01-HC-35129, N01-HC-15103, N01-HC-55222, N01-HC-75150, N01-HC-45133, and HHSN268201200036C, and NHLBI grants HL080295, HL087652, and HL105756 with additional contribution from NINDS. Additional support was provided through AG-023629, AG-15928, AG-20098, and AG-027058 from the NIA. See also http://www.chs-nhlbi.org/pi.htm. DNA handling and genotyping was supported in part by National Center of Advancing Translational Technologies CTSI grant UL1TR000124 and National Institute of Diabetes and Digestive and Kidney Diseases grant DK063491 to the Southern California Diabetes Endocrinology Research Center.

The content is solely the responsibility of the author and does not necessarily represent the official views of the National Institutes of Health.

## Further Reading

Balding, D.J. (2006) A tutorial on statistical methods for population association studies. *Nature Reviews Genetics* 7, 781–791.

Bouaziz, M., Ambroise, C. and Guedj, M. (2011) Accounting for population stratification in practice: a comparison of the main strategies dedicated to genome-wide association studies. *PloS One* 6, e28845.

Kang, H.M., Sul, J.H., Zaitlen, N.A., Kong, S., Freimer, N.B., Sabatti C., *et al.* (2010) Variance component model to account for sample structure in genome-wide association studies. *Nature Genetics* 42, 348–354.

Lemaitre, R.N., Tanaka, T., Tang, W., Manichaikul, A., Foy, M., Kabagambe, E.K., *et al.* (2011) Genetic loci associated with plasma phospholipid n-3 fatty acids: a meta-analysis of genome-wide association studies from the CHARGE Consortium. *PLoS Genetics* 7, e1002193.

Novembre, J., Johnson, T., Bryc, K., Kutalik, Z., Boyko, A.R., Auton, A., *et al.* (2008) Genes mirror geography within Europe. *Nature* 456, 98–101.

Price A.L., Zaitlen N.A., Reich D. and Patterson N. (2010) New approaches to population stratification in genome-wide association studies. *Nature Reviews Genetics* 11, 459–463.

Pritchard, J.K., Price, A.L., Tandon, A., Patterson, N., Barnes, K.C., Rafaels, N., *et al.* (2009) Sensitive detection of chromosomal segments of distinct ancestry in admixed populations. *PLoS Genetics* 5, e1000519.

Risch, N. and Merikangas, K. (1996) The future of genetic studies of complex human diseases. *Science* 273, 1516–1517.

## References

Alexander, D.H. and Lange, K. (2011) Enhancements to the admixture algorithm for individual ancestry estimation. *BMC Bioinformatics* 12, 246.

Alexander, D.H., Novembre, J. and Lange, K. (2009) Fast model-based estimation of ancestry in unrelated individuals. *Genome Research* 19, 1655–1664.

Bonnen, P.E., Lowe, J.K., Altshuler, D.M., Breslow, J.L., Stoffel, M., Friedman, J.M. and Pe'er I. (2009) European admixture on the Micronesian island of Kosrae: lessons from complete genetic information. *European Journal of Human Genetics* 18, 309–316.

Bouaziz, M., Ambroise, C. and Guedj, M. (2011) Accounting for population stratification in practice: a comparison of the main strategies dedicated to genome-wide association studies. *PloS One* 6, e28845.

Burton, P.R., Clayton, D.G., Cardon, L.R., Craddock, N., Deloukas, P., Duncanson, A., *et al.* (2007) Genome-wide association study of 14,000 cases of seven common diseases and 3,000 shared controls. *Nature* 447, 661–678.

Campbell, C.D., Ogburn, E.L., Lunetta, K.L., Lyon, H.N., Freedman, M.L., Groop, L.C., *et al.* (2005) Demonstrating stratification in a European American population. *Nature Genetics* 37, 868–872.

Carr, D.B., Littlefield, R.J., Nicholson, W.L., Littlefield, J.S. (1987) Scatterplot matrix techniques for large N. *Journal of the American Statistical Association* 82, 424–436.

Choi, Y., Wijsman, E.M. and Weir, B.S. (2009) Case–control association testing in the presence of unknown relationships. *Genetic Epidemiology* 33, 668–678.

Devlin, B. and Roeder, K. (1999) Genomic control for association studies. *Biometrics* 55, 997–1004.

Falush, D., Stephens, M. and Pritchard, J.K. (2003) Inference of population structure using multilocus genotype data: linked loci and correlated allele frequencies. *Genetics* 164, 1567–1587.

Kang, H.M., Sul, J.H., Zaitlen, N.A., Kong, S., Freimer, N.B., Sabatti, C. and Eskin, E. (2010) Variance component model to account for sample structure in genome-wide association studies. *Nature Genetics* 42, 348–354.

Koepsell, T.D. and Weiss, N.S. (2003) *Epidemiologic Methods: Studying the Occurrence of Illness.* Oxford University Press, New York, pp. 247–269.

Kullo, I.J., Ding, K., Shameer, K., McCarty, C.A., Jarvik, G.P., Denny, J.C., *et al.* (2011) Complement receptor 1 gene variants are associated with erythrocyte sedimentation rate. *American Journal of Human Genetics* 89, 131–138.

Lemaitre, R.N., Tanaka, T., Tang, W., Manichaikul, A., Foy, M., Kabagambe, E.K., *et al.* (2011) Genetic loci associated with plasma phospholipid n-3 fatty acids: a meta-analysis of genome-wide association studies from the CHARGE Consortium. *PLoS Genetics* 7, e1002193.

Li, J.Z., Absher, D.M., Tang, H., Southwick, A.M., Casto, A.M., Ramachandran, S., *et al.* (2008) Worldwide human relationships inferred from genome-wide patterns of variation. *Science* 319, 1100–1104.

Marchini, J., Cardon, L.R., Phillips, M.S. and Donnelly, P. (2004) The effects of human population structure on large genetic association studies. *Nature Genetics* 36, 512–517.

Novembre, J., Johnson, T., Bryc, K., Kutalik, Z., Boyko, A.R., Auton, A., *et al.* (2008) Genes mirror geography within Europe. *Nature* 456, 98–101.

Peloso, G. and Lunetta, K. (2011) Choice of population structure informative principal components for adjustment in a case–control study. *BMC Genetics* 12, 64.

Price, A.L., Patterson, N.J., Plenge, R.M., Weinblatt, M.E., Shadick, N.A. and Reich, D. (2006) Principal components analysis corrects for stratification in genome-wide association studies. *Nature Genetics* 38, 904–909.

Price, A.L., Zaitlen, N.A., Reich, D. and Patterson, N. (2010) New approaches to population stratification in genome-wide association studies. *Nature Reviews Genetics* 11, 459–463.

Pritchard, J.K., Stephens, M. and Donnelly, P. (2000) Inference of population structure using multilocus genotype data. *Genetics* 155, 945–959.

Pritchard, J.K., Price, A.L., Tandon, A., Patterson, N., Barnes, K.C., Rafaels, N., *et al.* (2009) Sensitive detection of chromosomal segments of distinct ancestry in admixed populations. *PLoS Genetics* 5, e1000519.

Qin, H., Morris, N., Kang, S.J., Li, M., Tayo, B., Lyon, H., *et al.* (2010) Interrogating local population structure for fine mapping in genome-wide association studies. *Bioinformatics* 26, 2961–2968.

Reiner, A.P., Lettre, G., Nalls, M.A., Ganesh, S.K., Mathias, R., Austin, M.A., *et al.* (2011) Genome-wide association study of white blood cell count in 16,388 African Americans: the Continental Origins and Genetic Epidemiology Network (COGENT). *PLoS Genetics* 7, e1002108.

Risch, N. and Merikangas, K. (1996) The future of genetic studies of complex human diseases. *Science* 273, 1516–1517.

Sabatti, C. (2008) Genome-wide association analysis of metabolic traits in a birth cohort from a founder population. *Nature Genetics* 41, 35–46.

Sladek, R., Rocheleau, G., Rung, J., Dina, C., Shen, L., Serre, D., *et al.* (2007) A genome-wide association study identifies novel risk loci for type 2 diabetes. *Nature* 445, 881–885.

Tang, H., Peng, J., Wang, P. and Risch, N.J. (2005) Estimation of individual admixture: analytical and study design considerations. *Genetic Epidemiology* 28, 289–301.

Tang, H., Choudhry, S., Mei, R., Morgan, M., Rodriguez-Cintron, W., Burchard, E.G. and Risch, N.J. (2007) Recent genetic selection in the ancestral admixture of Puerto Ricans. *American Journal of Human Genetics* 81, 626–633.

Thomas, G., Jacobs, K.B., Kraft, P., Yeager, M., Wacholder, S., Cox, D.G., *et al.* (2009) A multi-stage genome-wide association study in breast cancer identifies two new risk alleles at 1p11. 2 and 14q24. 1 (RAD51L1). *Nature Genetics* 41, 579–584.

Thornton, T. and McPeek, M.S. (2007) Case–control association testing with related individuals: a more powerful quasi-likelihood score test. *American Journal of Human Genetics* 81, 321–337.

Thornton, T. and McPeek, M.S. (2010) ROADTRIPS: case–control association testing with partially or completely unknown population and pedigree structure. *American Journal of Human Genetics* 86, 172–184.

Wang, X., Zhu, X., Qin, H., Cooper, R.S., Ewens, W.J., Li, C. and Li, M. (2011) Adjustment for local ancestry in genetic association analysis of admixed populations. *Bioinformatics* 27, 670–677.

Winkelmann, J., Czamara, D., Schormair, B., Knauf, F., Schulte, E.C., Trenkwalder, C., *et al.* (2011) Genome-wide association study identifies novel restless legs syndrome susceptibility loci on 2p14 and 16q12. 1. *PLoS Genetics* 7, e1002171.

Wu, C., DeWan, A., Hoh, J. and Wang, Z. (2011) A comparison of association methods correcting for population stratification in case–control studies. *Annals of Human Genetics* 75, 418–427.

## Web Resources

All web resources accessed on November 9, 2012.

ADMIXTURE software available at: http://www.genetics.ucla.edu/software/admixture
EIGENSOFT software available at: http://genepath.med.harvard.edu/~reich/Software.htm
EMMAX software available at: http://genetics.cs.ucla.edu/emmax/
FRAPPE software available at: http://med.stanford.edu/tanglab/software/frappe.html
HAPMIX software available at: http://www.stats.ox.ac.uk/~myers/software.html
Hexbin R package available at: http://cran.r-project.org/web/packages/hexbin/index.html
R software available at: http://www.r-project.org/
ROADTRIPS software available at: http://www.stat.uchicago.edu/~mcpeek/software/ROADTRIPS/index.html
STRUCTURE software available at: http://pritch.bsd.uchicago.edu/structure.html

# 7 Gene–Environment Interactions and Epistasis

MELISSA A. AUSTIN, M.S., PH.D.[1]
AND RUTH OTTMAN, PH.D.[2]

[1]Department of Epidemiology, University of Washington, Seattle, Washington; [2]G.H. Sergievsky Center and Departments of Epidemiology and Neurology, Columbia University, New York

## Synopsis

- Understanding gene–environment and gene–gene interactions (epistasis) can increase the statistical power, accuracy, and precision for detecting genetic and environmental effects, as well as improving our understanding of biological mechanisms of disease risk.
- Five biologically plausible models of relationships between a genotype and an exposure and their effect on disease risk are presented to conceptualize different types of interaction.
- The use of an additive or multiplicative measurement scale in evaluating interaction has important implications for the interpretation of interactions, and causal modeling approaches from epidemiology can be used to address this problem.
- The case-only study design is useful for evaluating interactions and can have higher statistical power than the standard case–control method, although it relies on the assumption that genetic and environmental risk factors occur independently and can only test for interaction on a multiplicative scale.
- One of the most important areas for the study of gene–environment interaction is pharmacogenomics, the study of the genetic bases for variation in drug response.
- Using genome-wide association study (GWAS) results combined with harmonized environmental data is an emerging approach for identifying gene–environment interactions and for discovering new genetic susceptibility variants.
- Taking into account epistasis is also important for understanding genetic pathways, and may improve the detection of genetic influences on complex diseases, including in the context of GWAS.

## 7.1 Why Study Interaction?

The study of gene–environment and gene–gene interactions is extremely important in genetic epidemiology, for a number of reasons. Understanding these interactions can increase power, accuracy, and precision in the detection of both genetic and environmental effects. Equally important, clarifying gene–environment and gene–gene interactions can improve our understanding of biological mechanisms and pathways for disease risk (Phillips, 2008; Thomas, 2010), which could, in turn, lead to the development of improved treatments or preventive measures. As described in Section 2.3.3, gene–environment or gene–gene interactions could explain some of the "missing heritability" in genome-wide association studies (GWAS) that may not be detected by marginal effects of single nucleotide polymorphisms (SNPs) associated with disease (Manolio *et al.*, 2009; Zuk *et al.*, 2012). Identifying gene–environment interactions may reveal environmental factors that affect only a subgroup of genetically susceptible individuals, with implications for targeted interventions to reduce modifiable risk factors in specific groups (Thomas, 2010). Ultimately, a better understanding of interactions will help refine public health recommendations for screening and intervention strategies.

In this chapter, we first consider five plausible models for gene–environment interactions. Then we discuss the problem of measurement scale for assessing interactions, and causal modeling approaches from epidemiology that have been used to inform selection of appropriate scales. We describe the case-only study design, using examples related to cardiovascular disease. We illustrate the emerging field of pharmacogenomics, the discovery of genotypes that influence efficacy or side effects of medications, with the example of carbamazepine and Stevens–Johnson syndrome. New developments in using GWAS results combined with harmonized environmental data to detect gene–environment interactions will be described. Finally, we define and discuss the concept of epistasis.

This overview will illustrate that interaction is a complex concept with both statistical and biological interpretations. Effective new methods are, however, being developed to detect gene–environment interactions that make use of standard epidemiologic study designs. Developments such as these will be central for both understanding disease mechanisms and developing effective methods to prevent and reduce disease risk in populations (Institute of Medicine, 2006).

## 7.2 Models of Interaction

From a statistical point of view, gene–environment interaction can be defined as a difference in the magnitude or direction of effect of an environmental exposure on disease risk in people with different genotypes, or, equivalently, a difference in the effect of a genotype on disease risk in people with different environmental exposures. As we discuss below, the problem of measurement scale arises from different interpretations of what is meant by a "difference" in these effects.

Figure 7.1 shows five biologically plausible models of relationships between a genotype and an exposure in their effect on disease risk, where both genotype and exposure are simple dichotomous variables (Ottman, 1990, 1996). Here we discuss each of these models briefly, and provide examples considering the (hypothetical) effects of a genotype and dietary fat on the risk of obesity.

In Model A, the genotype does not have a direct effect on disease risk, but instead increases expression of a factor generally considered to be an "environmental exposure." For example, a genotype associated with appetite control might lead to increased consumption of dietary fat and consequently raise the risk of obesity. From an epidemiologic point of view, this is actually a model of *mediation* rather than interaction – dietary fat is an intervening variable between the genotype (exposure)

M.A. Austin and R. Ottman

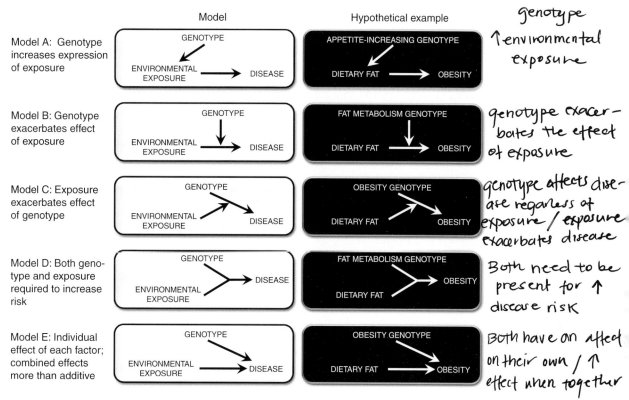

Model | Hypothetical example

Model A: Genotype increases expression of exposure — GENOTYPE → ENVIRONMENTAL EXPOSURE → DISEASE | APPETITE-INCREASING GENOTYPE → DIETARY FAT → OBESITY

*genotype ↑ environmental exposure*

Model B: Genotype exacerbates effect of exposure — GENOTYPE ↓ ENVIRONMENTAL EXPOSURE → DISEASE | FAT METABOLISM GENOTYPE ↓ DIETARY FAT → OBESITY

*genotype exacer- bates the effect of exposure*

Model C: Exposure exacerbates effect of genotype — GENOTYPE / ENVIRONMENTAL EXPOSURE → DISEASE | OBESITY GENOTYPE / DIETARY FAT → OBESITY

*genotype affects dise- are regarless of exposure / exposure exacerbates disease*

Model D: Both geno- type and exposure required to increase risk — GENOTYPE / ENVIRONMENTAL EXPOSURE → DISEASE | FAT METABOLISM GENOTYPE / DIETARY FAT → OBESITY

*Both need to be present for ↑ discase risk*

Model E: Individual effect of each factor; combined effects more than additive — GENOTYPE / ENVIRONMENTAL EXPOSURE → DISEASE | OBESITY GENOTYPE / DIETARY FAT → OBESITY

*Both have an affect on their own / ↑ effect when together*

**Fig. 7.1.** Five models of relationships between a genotype and environmental risk factor in their effects on disease risk, described by Ottman (1990, 1996).

and the outcome (obesity). Although this does not meet the definition of interaction above, we include it here because it is an important model of relationships between genes and exposures; if the factors that intervene between a genotype and its disease-raising effects could be elucidated, we might ultimately be able to reduce or eliminate some genetic effects on disease risk.

In Model B, the exposure has a direct effect on disease regardless of whether or not the genotype is present. The genotype has no effect on disease when the exposure is absent, but it exacerbates the effect of the exposure when it is present. In the obes-ity example, we might imagine a genotype that affects fat metabolism, so that the effect of dietary fat on obesity is greater when the genotype is present, but there is no effect of the genotype in the absence of dietary fat.

Model C is the converse of Model B. Here, the genotype affects disease risk regardless of whether or not the exposure is present. The exposure has no effect in the absence of the genotype, but exacerbates disease risk when the genotype is present. In the obesity example, we would postulate an obesity-related genotype that affects risk regardless of diet, but whose effect is worsened in individuals who con-sume high amounts of fat. Under this model, individuals who eat fat but do not have the genotype would not have increased risk of obesity.

In Model D, there is no effect of either genotype or exposure unless both are present. In the obesity example, this would be a situation where a genotype affects risk only in individuals who eat fat, and a diet with high amounts of fat has no effect on obesity in individuals without this genotype.

Finally, in Model E, each of the factors – genotype and exposure – has an effect on risk when acting by itself, but when both are present the effect is greater than expected based on the combined influence of the two factors. This is the situation where it is crucial to define the measurement scale, because different measurement scales lead to different predictions about the expected combined effect of the two factors.

Table 7.1 summarizes the pattern of disease relative risk expected with each of these models, in individuals with each of the four possible combinations of a dichotomous genotype and dichotomous exposure. In the table, individuals with neither the high-risk genotype nor the exposure are used as the reference category (shown as relative risk "1"), and for each of the other categories, "+" indicates an increased risk is expected, and "++" indicates a greater increase in risk is expected. Because all of these patterns are different, the five models in Fig. 7.1 can be distinguished from each other if data are available on a dichotomous genotype and exposure.

Under certain simplifying assumptions, Models B, C, D, and E form a comprehensive set of possible models of gene–environment interaction. The simplifying assumptions are: (i) each factor (genotype or exposure) is a simple dichotomous trait; (ii) both factors are associated with increased, rather than decreased, risk; and (iii) interactions are synergistic, rather than antagonistic. Under these assumptions, there are four possible models, defined by whether each of the two factors does or does not raise disease risk in the absence of the other: exposure only (Model B), genotype only (Model C), neither (Model D), or both (Model E), with synergy of the effects assumed in each case. If we were to expand the list to consider factors with either risk-raising or protective effects, each of the two factors could have either a risk-raising effect, a protective effect, or no effect in the absence of the other, for a total of $3 \times 3 = 9$ possible combinations; and if we consider possible antagonism in addition to synergy (e.g. a genotype suppresses the effect of an exposure), we have even more possibilities for interaction. This illustrates the complexity of evaluating interactions, even for a single

**Table 7.1.** Patterns of risk in different models.

| Model | High-risk genotype present | | High-risk genotype absent | |
|---|---|---|---|---|
| | Exposure present | Exposure absent | Exposure present | Exposure absent |
| **A.** Genotype increases expression of risk factor | + | 1 | + | 1 |
| **B.** Genotype exacerbates the effect of exposure | ++ | 1 | + | 1 |
| **C.** Exposure exacerbates the effect of genotype | ++ | + | 1 | 1 |
| **D.** Both genotype and exposure required to increase risk | + | 1 | 1 | 1 |
| **E.** Genotype and exposure each affect risk; combined effects greater than additive | ++ | + | + | 1 |

M.A. Austin and R. Ottman

dichotomized genotype and a single dichotomous environmental exposure. Analysis of variations in quantitative responses to risk factors is also not considered here.

## 7.3 Statistical Interaction and the Problem of Measurement Scale

In this section, statistical approaches to defining gene–environment interactions are developed. In general, an interaction is present when the effect of an exposure varies according to genotype or the effect of genotype varies by exposure, i.e. in epidemiologic terms, when there is *effect modification* (Knol and VanderWeele, 2012). Although this seems to be simple definition, detecting the presence of interaction depends on what is meant by a "different effect," which in turn depends on the measurement scale used in the analysis.

### 7.3.1 Statistical analysis of interaction for cohort and case–control studies

To illustrate the statistical concepts of interaction, we begin with analysis of a cohort study in which individuals are classified by a high-risk genotype and a high-risk environmental exposure, and disease risks are evaluated in the four resulting groups. Table 7.2 shows how we would calculate the disease risk in each group of individuals in this case.

To evaluate gene–environment interaction, we are interested in determining whether or not the effect of the exposure differs among people with and without the genotype. There are (at least) two different ways we can evaluate the effect of the exposure. First, we could compute the *relative risk* (RR) in individuals with (G+) and without (G–) the genotype: $RR_{G+} = r_{11}/r_{01}$ and $RR_{G-} = r_{10}/r_{00}$. Ratio measures such as the RR assess risks on a *multiplicative* scale, i.e. they assess how much the risk in one group is *multiplied* in order to obtain the risk in the other.

**Table 7.2.** Data layout for cohort study of gene–environment interaction.

| Disease outcome | High-risk genotype present | | High-risk genotype absent | |
|---|---|---|---|---|
| | Exposure present | Exposure absent | Exposure present | Exposure absent |
| Affected | a | b | e | f |
| Unaffected | c | d | g | h |
| Disease risk estimate | $r_{11} = a/(a+c)$ | $r_{01} = b/(b+d)$ | $r_{10} = e/(e+g)$ | $r_{00} = f/(f+h)$ |
| Measure of exposure effect within genotype strata: | | | | |
| Multiplicative scale | $RR_{G+} = r_{11}/r_{01}$ | | $RR_{G-} = r_{10}/r_{00}$ | |
| Additive scale | $RD_{G+} = r_{11}-r_{01}$ | | $RD_{G-} = r_{10}-r_{00}$ | |
| RR with common referent | $RR_{G+E+} = r_{11}/r_{00}$ | $RR_{G+E-} = r_{01}/r_{00}$ | $RR_{G-E+} = r_{10}/r_{00}$ | $RR_{G-E-} = r_{00}/r_{00} = 1$ (reference) |

Alternatively, we could compute the *risk difference* (RD) in the two genotype groups: $RD_{G+} = r_{11} - r_{01}$ and $RD_{G-} = r_{10} - r_{00}$. The RD assesses risk on an *additive* scale, i.e. it assesses how much risk is *added* to the risk in one group in order to obtain the risk in the other.

The different measurement scales have extremely important implications for the interpretation of whether or not interaction is present. If we measure risk on a multiplicative scale, we would say there is no interaction if the two RRs are the same (i.e. $RR_{G+} = RR_{G-}$), whereas if we measure risk on an additive scale, we would say there is no interaction if the two RDs are the same (i.e. $RD_{G+} = RD_{G-}$). The only conditions under which both of these two criteria can be met are when there is no effect of the genotype in the absence of the exposure (i.e. $r_{01} = r_{00}$), there is no effect of the exposure in the absence of the genotype (i.e. $r_{10} = r_{00}$), or both. (Note that these conditions are met for Models B, C, and D described above – so that interaction is present regardless of which scale is used. For Model E, however, conclusions about whether or not interaction is present depend on which measurement scale is used.)

Table 7.2 also shows a different type of RR, defined for each of the groups using individuals with neither genotype nor exposure as a common reference category ($RR_{G+E+}$, $RR_{G+E-}$, $RR_{G-E+}$, and the referent, $RR_{G-E-}$). These RRs are convenient because they can be used to evaluate interaction on either a multiplicative or an additive scale. This is because, by simple algebra, it can be shown that:

$$RR_{G+} = RR_{G-} \text{ (no interaction on a multiplicative scale)} \Rightarrow RR_{G+E+} = RR_{G+E-} \times RR_{G-E+}$$

and

$$RD_{G+} = RD_{G-} \text{ (no interaction on an additive scale)} \Rightarrow RR_{G+E+} = RR_{G+E-} + RR_{G-E+} - 1$$

As discussed below, these relationships are especially useful for case–control studies, where risks and RD cannot be estimated, and odds ratios (ORs) are used to estimate RRs.

Table 7.3 shows the data layout for a case–control study of gene–environment interaction, according to the "two-by-four" format proposed by Botto and Khoury (2001) that contains the number of cases and controls with each possible combination of the high-risk genotype and a dichotomized environmental risk factor. Analogous to the RRs described above for cohort studies, four ORs are calculated, with the cases and controls with neither the high-risk genotype nor the environmental risk factor (g, h) used as the reference category. Standard methods can be used to test the statistical significance of the ORs and to determine confidence intervals.

This table provides a clear and complete display of the primary data and allows comparisons of the combined effects of genotype and environmental exposure with the effects of genotype alone and environmental exposure alone under different measurement scales (see Section 7.3.2). It also allows estimates of the OR for case-only studies (see Section 7.4) (Botto and Khoury, 2001). However, the simplifying assumption of dichotomizing the environment exposure must be kept in mind because "dose" of environmental exposure is important for many risk factors, such as smoking or drinking alcohol, for example.

M.A. Austin and R. Ottman

**Table 7.3.** Case–control study layout for analysis of gene–environment interaction (adapted from Botto and Khoury, 2001).

|  | High-risk genotype present | | High-risk genotype absent | |
| --- | --- | --- | --- | --- |
|  | Exposure present | Exposure absent | Exposure present | Exposure absent |
| Cases | a | c | e | g |
| Controls | b | d | f | h |
| ORs | $OR_{G+E+} = ah/bg$ | $OR_{G+E-} = ch/dg$ | $OR_{G-E+} = eh/fg$ | 1.0 (reference) |

### 7.3.2 Multiplicative and additive measurement scales

Once these RRs and ORs are available, the determination of whether or not interaction is present depends on whether a multiplicative or additive scale is used. Table 7.4 shows the expectations for no interaction, synergistic interaction, and antagonistic interaction, in cohort and case–control studies, as a function of the scale of measurement used for assessment. Here we define synergistic interaction as a *greater* effect of the exposure in individuals with the high-risk genotype than in individuals with the low-risk genotype, and antagonism as a *smaller* effect of the exposure in individuals with the high-risk genotype than in those with the low-risk genotype. The formulas shown for the ORs are only approximations, but should be reasonable if the ORs are reasonable estimates of the RRs.

We noted above that the only conditions under which the expectations of no interaction are met under both the additive and multiplicative models are when there is no effect of one or both factors in the absence of the other. Examination of Table 7.4 illustrates that, under these special conditions, the expectations are the same not only for no interaction, but also for synergy and antagonism. For example, if $RR_{G+E-} = 1$ (i.e. no effect of the genotype in the absence of the exposure), the expectation of no interaction on a multiplicative scale is $RR_{G+E+} = 1 \times RR_{G-E+} = RR_{G-E+}$. The expectation of no interaction on an additive scale is the same: $RR_{G+E+} = 1 + RR_{G-E+} - 1 = RR_{G-E+}$. Similarly, if $RR_{G+E-} = 1$, the expectation under synergy is $RR_{G+E+} > RR_{G-E+}$, and the expectation under antagonism is $RR_{G+E+} < RR_{G-E+}$, under either the multiplicative or additive model. Similar results apply to the ORs, assuming they are reasonable estimates of the RRs.

However, if neither $RR_{G+E-} = 1$ nor $RR_{G-E+} = 1$, the expectations under the additive and multiplicative scales will always differ. Moreover, because the expectations of *no interaction* are different under the two measurement scales, a finding of no interaction on one scale will always indicate interaction on the other. For example, suppose the findings of a study showed that $OR_{G+E-}$ and $OR_{G-E+}$ are both equal to 3. If a multiplicative scale were used to assess interaction, the investigators would conclude there is no interaction if $OR_{G+E+} = 3 \times 3 = 9$, but if they used an additive scale, they would conclude there is no interaction if $OR_{G+E+} = 3 + 3 - 1 = 5$. Hence a finding that $OR_{G+E+} = 9$ would indicate no interaction on a multiplicative scale, but synergy on an additive scale.

To make matters even more complicated, a simple mathematical transformation of the data (e.g. to a logistic scale) could be made, and the findings regarding interaction – even if the same scale were used – could differ between the transformed and untransformed data. For example, one of the most common ways to test for interaction in epidemiology

**Table 7.4.** Expectations for no interaction, synergy, and antagonism in cohort and case–control studies, using different measurement scales.

| Measurement scale and interaction effect | Cohort study | Case–control study[a] |
|---|---|---|
| **Multiplicative scale** | | |
| No interaction | $RR_{G+E+} = RR_{G+E-} \times RR_{G-E+}$ | $OR_{G+E+} = OR_{G+E-} \times OR_{G-E+}$ |
| Synergistic interaction | $RR_{G+E+} > RR_{G+E-} \times RR_{G-E+}$ | $OR_{G+E+} > OR_{G+E-} \times OR_{G-E+}$ |
| Antagonistic interaction | $RR_{G+E+} < RR_{G+E-} \times RR_{G-E+}$ | $OR_{G+E+} < OR_{G+E-} \times OR_{G-E+}$ |
| **Additive scale** | | |
| No interaction | $RR_{G+E+} = RR_{G+E-} + RR_{G-E+} - 1$ | $OR_{G+E+} = OR_{G+E-} + OR_{G-E+} - 1$ |
| Synergistic interaction | $RR_{G+E+} > RR_{G+E-} + RR_{G-E+} - 1$ | $OR_{G+E+} > OR_{G+E-} + OR_{G-E+} - 1$ |
| Antagonistic interaction | $RR_{G+E+} < RR_{G+E-} + RR_{G-E+} - 1$ | $OR_{G+E+} < OR_{G+E-} + OR_{G-E+} - 1$ |

[a]Formulas for the ORs are approximations based on the approximation of the OR to the RR.

is to add an interaction term to a logistic regression model. This is a test of interaction of the lnORs on an additive scale – that is, in the context of gene–environment interaction, it tests for a significant deviation from the expectation that:

$$\ln OR_{G+E+} = (\ln OR_{G+E-} + \ln OR_{G-E+})$$

If we convert this back to the scale of ORs (rather than lnORs), we have:

$$\ln OR_{G+E+} = (\ln OR_{G+E-} + \ln OR_{G-E+}) = \ln(OR_{G+E-} \times OR_{G-E+}), \text{ which implies:}$$

$$OR_{G+E+} = (OR_{G+E-} \times OR_{G-E+})$$

i.e. a test of multiplicativity of the ORs!

### 7.3.3 Causal modeling applied to interaction

The different expectations under the additive and multiplicative models point to a critical problem in the assessment of gene–environment interaction. Investigators using different scales to measure interaction would reach different conclusions about whether or not interaction is present. The different possible interpretations are potentially very serious, because medical or public health interventions could be initiated based on the conclusions.

Which measurement scale *should* we use to test for interaction? In many epidemiologic analyses, the decision is primarily based on convenience – a multiplicative scale is used because the analytic approaches (e.g. logistic regression) and statistical packages used to implement them (e.g. SAS, SPSS) routinely test for interaction on a multiplicative, rather than an additive, scale. This is, however, clearly not the best way to decide which scale is most appropriate!

Epidemiologists have approached this problem by using reasoning based on causal, rather than purely statistical, models. Unlike many statistical models used in genetic epidemiology, causal models are explicitly formulated in terms of cause and effect relationships occurring at the *individual* level (Madsen *et al.*, 2011a). Statistics and measurement scales are not relevant when we consider this individual response, and hence causal modeling provides an entirely different way to approach the problem that is

M.A. Austin and R. Ottman

more closely tied to disease mechanisms. The conclusion based on this reasoning is that the *additive scale* is the most appropriate one to use to test for interaction. It has also been noted that additive interaction is appropriate for public health applications because it reflects disease burden in the population (Thomas, 2010).

In one of the most prominent causal modeling frameworks, sufficient-component cause modeling (Rothman and Greenland, 1998), a *sufficient cause* is defined as "a set of minimal conditions and events that inevitably produce disease," and a *component cause* as one of the minimal conditions or events included in a sufficient cause. In this framework, two factors "interact" (in a biological sense) if they are components of the same sufficient cause. Hence gene–environment interaction would be defined as a mechanism of disease causation (i.e. a sufficient cause) in which both a genotype and an environmental exposure are necessary. In addition, the sufficient-component cause framework assumes that multiple sufficient causes are involved in the cause of a given disease, so that some individuals develop disease in the absence of either genotype or environmental exposure.

In this conceptualization, a test for gene–environment interaction would involve evaluating whether there are any sufficient causes of disease that involve both a genotype and an environmental exposure. To develop such a test, we use another causal modeling approach, potential outcomes theory (Greenland and Robins, 1986; Greenland and Robins, 2009; Madsen *et al.*, 2011a). In this framework, "response types" are classes defined by the potential outcomes an individual could demonstrate if exposed to a given set of risk factors. For a dichotomous genotype and a dichotomous exposure, theoretically there are 16 possible response types (i.e. affected or unaffected for each of the four possible combinations, or $2 \times 2 \times 2 \times 2 = 16$). However, if we make the simple and reasonable assumption that the same factor cannot both cause and prevent disease, the list of possible response types is reduced to 6, as illustrated in Table 7.5.

Table 7.5 assigns a name to each of the six response types and indicates whether individuals with that type are affected or unaffected when they have each combination of genotype and exposure. The first response type is called "inevitable" (sometimes also called "doomed") (Greenland and Robins, 1986), because people in this category

**Table 7.5.** Potential outcomes for a dichotomous genotype and exposure.

| Response type | High-risk genotype | | Low-risk genotype | | Proportion of individuals with response type |
|---|---|---|---|---|---|
| | Exposed | Unexposed | Exposed | Unexposed | |
| Inevitable | Affected | Affected | Affected | Affected | $p_1$ |
| Gene susceptible | Affected | Affected | Unaffected | Unaffected | $p_2$ |
| Exposure susceptible | Affected | Unaffected | Affected | Unaffected | $p_3$ |
| Parallel | Affected | Affected | Affected | Unaffected | $p_4$ |
| Synergistic | Affected | Unaffected | Unaffected | Unaffected | $p_5$ |
| Immune | Unaffected | Unaffected | Unaffected | Unaffected | $p_6$ |
| Population disease risk | $r_{11}$ | $r_{01}$ | $r_{10}$ | $r_{00}$ | |
| Proportion of individuals who are affected | $p_1+p_2+p_3$ $+p_4+p_5$ | $p_1+p_2+p_4$ | $p_1+p_3+p_4$ | $p_1$ | |

will be affected regardless of whether or not they have the genotype or exposure. People with the second response type, "gene susceptible," will be affected if they have the genotype regardless of whether or not they have the exposure. People with the third type, "exposure susceptible," will be affected if exposed, regardless of their genotype. People with the fourth type, "parallel," will be affected if they have either the genotype or the exposure; it doesn't matter whether or not they have both. The fifth type is "synergistic": people in this category will be affected only if they have both genotype and exposure. Finally, the sixth type, "immune," consists of individuals who will never be affected regardless of whether they have the genotype or exposure.

This conceptualization of response types in individuals also allows us to predict average risks in the population. The column on the right of Table 7.5 shows the proportion of individuals in the population with each response type. These proportions reflect the distribution of response types in the population, and are used to estimate population disease risk for each of the four genotype/exposure categories. This is done by summing, within each genotype/exposure category, the proportion of individuals with response types who are affected within that category. For example, among people with neither genotype nor exposure, only those with the "inevitable" response type will be affected, so the proportion of individuals who are affected in that category is $p_1$. Similarly, among people with the exposure but without the high-risk genotype, those with the "inevitable," "exposure susceptible," or "parallel" response types will be affected, so the proportion affected in that category is $p_1+p_3+p_4$.

To evaluate interaction, ideally we would like to know whether there are any individuals in the population of the "synergistic type," i.e. we would like to test the null hypothesis that $p_5 = 0$. We cannot test this hypothesis directly, but we can come close. In Table 7.2 above, we defined four "$r_{ij}$ values" corresponding to the disease risk in the four categories of genotype and exposure; these are also shown in Table 7.5, along with the estimates of average risk based on response types. The null hypothesis for the test for interaction on an additive scale is $RD_{G+} = RD_{G-}$, i.e. $(r_{11}-r_{01}) = (r_{01}-r_{00})$. In terms of the potential outcomes model, this is equivalent to:

$$(p_1+p_2+p_3+p_4+p_5) - (p_1+p_2+p_4) = (p_1+p_3+p_4) - p_1 \Rightarrow p_5 = p_4$$

This implies that a test for interaction on an additive scale is equivalent to a test for a difference in the frequency of synergistic and parallel types in the population. That is, it is a test of whether people who would develop disease only if exposed to *both* a high-risk genotype and an environmental exposure are more (or less) frequent than those who would develop disease if exposed to *either* one alone.

This seems to be a sensible way to think about whether or not there are sufficient causes that involve both a genotype and an environmental exposure. A test of interaction on a multiplicative scale would not be interpretable in this way, suggesting that the additive scale is the most meaningful metric for the measurement of interaction. Two caveats must be kept in mind, however. First, rejection of the hypothesis of no interaction on an additive scale does not necessarily imply synergistic types are more frequent than parallel types – they could also be less frequent. Secondly, failure to reject the hypothesis of no interaction on an additive scale does not necessarily imply there are no synergistic types in the population, because the synergistic and parallel types could balance each other out.

Although epidemiologists have generally reached agreement that the additive scale is preferable for testing for interaction (Rothman, 1976; VanderWeele and

M.A. Austin and R. Ottman

Robins, 2007), the statistical methods used most frequently in epidemiologic studies do not incorporate such tests. As discussed above, logistic regression tests for interaction on a multiplicative scale – and since the product of two ORs is generally greater than their sum minus 1, failure to find evidence for interaction in logistic regression does not exclude the possibility of interaction on an additive scale.

---

**Box 7.1. Application: Factor V Leiden**

One of the best examples of gene–environment interaction involves the Factor V Leiden variant (genetic factor), oral contraceptive (OC) use (environmental factor), and risk of deep vein thrombosis (DVT) (see Box 5.1 for background). This example is from a study of 155 pre-menopausal women who developed DVT and 169 population controls (Vandenbroucke *et al.*, 1994).

As illustrated in Table 7.6, $OR_{G-E+}$ the OR for DVT among women who use OCs but do not carry Factor V Leiden, = 3.7. A somewhat higher, and also statistically significant, increase in risk is seen among women with Factor V Leiden who do not take OCs: $OR_{G+E-} = 6.9$. However, the OR for DVT among women with Factor V Leiden who do use OCs is much higher: $OR_{G+E+} = 34.7$.

We can evaluate these ORs in terms of the multiplicative and additive scales described above. That is, for a multiplicative interaction, we compare $OR_{G+E+}$ with $OR_{G+E-} \times OR_{G-E+}$:

$$OR_{G+E+} = 34.7 \text{ and } OR_{G+E-} \times OR_{G-E+} = 6.9 \times 3.7 = 25.7$$

For additive interaction, we compare $OR_{G+E+}$ with $OR_{G+E-} + OR_{G-E+} - 1$:

$$OR_{G+E+} = 34.7 \text{ and } OR_{G+E-} + OR_{G-E+} - 1 = 6.9 + 3.7 - 1 = 9.6$$

We can see that $OR_{G+E+}$ (34.7) is somewhat higher than expected under a multiplicative scale (25.7), but the difference is not too great, especially given the wide confidence interval for $OR_{G+E+}$. In contrast, $OR_{G+E+}$ (34.7) is considerably larger than expected under an additive scale (9.6). Thus this example provides evidence for synergy on an additive scale, but does not provide evidence for interaction on a multiplicative scale. It also illustrates that the determination of whether or not interaction is present depends on the chosen statistical scale and, more generally that investigators using different scales to analyze the same data would reach different conclusions about whether or not interaction is present.

**Table 7.6.** ORs for statistical evaluation of gene–environment interactions (adapted from Vandenbroucke *et al.*, 1994; Botto and Khoury, 2001).

| | Factor V Leiden present | | Factor V Leiden absent | |
|---|---|---|---|---|
| | OC use | | OC use | |
| | Present | Absent | Present | Absent |
| Cases | 25 | 10 | 84 | 36 |
| Controls | 2 | 4 | 63 | 100 |
| ORs | $OR_{G+E+} = 34.7$ | $OR_{G+E-} = 6.9$ | $OR_{G-E+} = 3.7$ | 1.0 |
| 95% confidence interval | (7.8, 310.0) | (1.83, 31.6) | (1.3, 6.3) | (reference) |

---

At the present time, most statistical packages easily measure interaction only on a multiplicative scale, making comparisons between multiplicative and additive scales difficult, especially in multivariate analyses. However, several statistics have been proposed for interaction tests on an additive scale, such as the relative excess risk due to interaction (RERI), the proportion attributable to interaction (AP), and the synergy index (S) (Rothman and Greenland, 1998). Thus, for example, rather than simply including an interaction term in the logistic regression model (which would test for interaction on a multiplicative scale), a test for interaction on an additive scale can be carried out by computing the RERI and its associated confidence interval (Richardson and Kaufman, 2009).

## 7.4   Case-only Study Design

The case-only design is another useful approach for evaluating interactions (Khoury and Flanders, 1996). Although this method cannot test for main effects of genotypes or environmental factors, it can have higher statistical power than the standard case–control method with the same number of cases (Yang *et al.*, 1997). The case-only design can be used if no controls are available for a study, or if limited resources allow only for genotyping of cases. However, this study design relies on the assumption that genetic and environmental risk factors occur independently in the source population, and there can be an increased false-positive rate if this assumption is violated (Thomas, 2010).

The case-only OR is a test of association between the genotype and the exposure within the cases only. Table 7.7 shows how the data from Table 7.3 are rearranged to perform this test.

The case-only OR is then calculated as:

Case-only OR = ag/ce

Departure of the case-only OR from 1 indicates the presence of interaction on a multiplicative scale, as described in Section 7.3. In the event that controls are available, the "control-only" OR can also be calculated from the data in Table 7.3 as:

Control-only OR = bh/df

If controls are thought to be representative of the source population, a control-only OR near 1 indicates independence of genetic and environmental factors, and thus provides a test of the underlying assumption of this study design. A case-only study is described in Box 7.2.

### 7.4.1   Considerations for case-only studies

Although the case-only method can be an efficient method for detecting interaction (Albert *et al.*, 2001), two important limitations of this approach should be kept in mind. First, as noted above, the case-only OR detects interaction on a multiplicative scale, and main effects cannot be evaluated. Secondly, the assumption of independence between the genotype and exposure is critical and inferences about the presence of multiplicative interaction can be distorted if there is departure from

**Table 7.7.** Data layout for case-only study of gene–environment interaction.

| | Cases with genotype | Cases without genotype |
|---|---|---|
| Exposed | a | e |
| Unexposed | c | g |

---

**Box 7.2. Application: Factor II, Hormone Replacement Therapy and Myocardial Infarction**

To illustrate the use of the case-only method, we will consider a study of the prothrombin G20210A variant, hormone replacement therapy, and risk of non-fatal myocardial infarction (MI) in the setting of a Group Health Cooperative in Seattle (Psaty *et al.*, 2001). The study was based on a sample of hypertensive post-menopausal women with a first non-fatal MI and frequency matched controls. Table 7.8 shows the results for the 108 cases and 385 controls with hypertension. For this analysis, the AA and AG genotypes were combined as the high-risk genotype and current hormone replacement therapy was the environmental factor.

The case-only OR = ag/ce = (6 × 65)/(2 × 35) = 5.6 with a 95% confidence interval of (1.1, 29.1). This significant finding indicates interaction on a multiplicative scale between the high-risk prothrombin variant and hormone replacement therapy on the risk of non-fatal MI among these hypertensive women.

Because controls are available from this study, they can be used to test the important assumption that the genotype and the exposure are independent. For the data in Table 7.8, the control-only OR = bh/df = (2 × 236)/(5 × 142) = 0.7. This value is near 1.0, providing evidence that the assumption is met.

**Table 7.8.** Study of the prothrombin variant G20210A, hormone replacement therapy, and non-fatal MI in women (adapted from Psaty *et al.*, 2001).

| | High-risk genotype (AA,AG) | | Low-risk genotype (GG) | |
|---|---|---|---|---|
| | Hormone therapy use | | Hormone therapy use | |
| | Present | Absent | Present | Absent |
| Non-fatal MI | 6 | 2 | 35 | 65 |
| Controls | 2 | 5 | 142 | 236 |

---

this assumption (Albert *et al.*, 2001). Examples of circumstances in which this assumption could be violated include diseases with a behavioral component, hormone-related cancers, non-randomized studies of treatment outcomes, and the presence of uncontrolled population stratification (Thomas *et al.*, 2012). If controls are not available, or are not representative of the source population, investigators can consider finding external data for this purpose, can explicitly test this assumption (Umbach and Weinberg, 1997), and/or can use adjustment procedures (Gatto *et al.*, 2004).

## 7.5 Pharmacogenomics

One of the most important areas for the study of gene–environment interaction is pharmacogenomics: the discovery of genotypes that influence efficacy or side effects of medications (Kasarskis *et al.*, 2011). This field has important implications for "personalized medicine" and public health, and to date has focused on approved prescription drugs (Giacomini *et al.*, 2012). The example discussed in Box 7.1 is a classic example of pharmacogenomics – an increased susceptibility to deep vein thrombosis as a consequence of oral contraceptive exposure, in women with the Factor V Leiden genetic variant.

Another more recent example is related to carbamazepine, a medication approved for the treatment of epilepsy, bipolar I disorders, trigeminal neuralgia, and more general neuropathic pain. Treatment with this drug is associated with serious and sometimes fatal dermatological reactions such as Stevens–Johnson syndrome (SJS) and toxic epidermal necrolysis (TEN). Researchers in Asia identified a strong association between inheritance of the HLA-B*1502 allele and SJS/TEN (Chung *et al.*, 2004). A recent study in Taiwan demonstrated the effectiveness of screening for HLA-B*1502 before treatment with carbamazepine, for the prevention of SJS/TEN (Chen *et al.*, 2011). The frequency of the HLA-B*1502 allele differs by ethnic group, and is highest in East Asia. In Europeans, carbamazepine sensitivity was found to be associated with another HLA allele, HLA-A*3101 (McCormack *et al.*, 2011). Because SJS also occurs in individuals treated with carbamazepine who do not have the HLA-B*1502 allele in Asia (though at much lower rates than in those with the allele), the findings are most consistent with Model B described in Section 7.2, where the genotype exacerbates the effect of the carbamazepine.

## 7.6 Gene–Environment-wide Interaction Studies (GEWIS)

The remarkable success of GWAS described in Chapter 5 creates unprecedented opportunities for studying the role of gene–environment interactions in disease risk by integrating associations found in GWAS with environmental risk factors (Khoury and Wacholder, 2009). These emerging types of studies have been termed gene–environment-wide interaction studies or GEWIS. They provide opportunities for both identifying gene–environment interactions by building on existing GWAS results and for discovering new SNP susceptibility variants that are not identified in studies that only consider marginal genetic effects.

Several ongoing challenges remain in order for these types of studies to be successful. Statistical power is generally low for interaction analyses compared with tests for main effects (Khoury and Wacholder, 2009). This necessitates enormous sample sizes, usually in the context of large-scale consortia, and thus requires the "harmonization" of environmental and behavioral variables, and the development of new statistical methods. As described briefly below, both of these areas are advancing rapidly.

### 7.6.1 Harmonization of environmental data

Harmonization of previously collected environmental data, usually from many collaborating studies, is one of the major challenges of GEWIS. Such environmental phenotypes have usually been obtained using different questionnaires and data

M.A. Austin and R. Ottman

collection methods that must be combined for data analysis. Further, unlike genomic data that are "static," environmental risk factors can change over time, and these variations may impact subsequent disease risk. Dealing with this phenotypic heterogeneity is essential for successfully identifying gene–environment interactions.

At least two projects have proposed systematic approaches to data harmonization: DataSchema and Harmonization Platform for Epidemiologic Research (DataSHaPER), intended for retrospective harmonization of data from large population-based studies (Fortier *et al.*, 2011), and the Phenotypes and eXposures (PhenX) Toolkit, "designed to provide a core set of well-established, low-burden, high-quality measures for use in large-scale genomic studies" (Hamilton *et al.*, 2011).

The DataSHaPER approach was developed to identify and document a set of core variables from collaborating studies and to assess their "inferential equivalence" based on existing information from individual studies. It uses a three-level scale of compatibility for assessing variables from participating studies, ranging from "complete" to "partial" to "impossible." In an analysis of 148 baseline variables from 53 large-scale studies over a long time span, 38% of the variables could be rigorously harmonized (Fortier *et al.*, 2011). Continuing development of this method, including extending it to longitudinal data, will be a valuable resource for data synthesis.

The PhenX project uses a consensus process involving a steering committee and working groups to identify a standard set of 15 measures in each of 21 research domains that can be used prospectively in studies collecting new data. The motivation for the identification of these common measures includes the recognition that many complex diseases have similar risk factors (smoking and diet, for example), standard measures will facilitate replication of GWAS results and enhanced statistical power from larger sample sizes and meta-analyses, and an accessible source of standard measures will allow investigators to expand the scope of their studies (Hamilton *et al.*, 2011).

Bennett *et al.* (2011) have recently illustrated the process of phenotype harmonization in the Gene–Environment Association Studies (GENEVA) GWAS Consortium, and suggest that it could facilitate the identification of new susceptibility loci for subtypes of disease and the characterization of shared variants among broad categories of diseases. These investigators describe a multistep process with the goal of maximizing the comparability of data and minimizing inconsistencies and misclassifications. The steps involved include:

1. Identifying common phenotypes.
2. Determining the feasibility of cross-study analyses.
3. Preparing common definitions.
4. Creating algorithms for coding and converting variables to a common format.
5. Drafting a data analysis plan for cross-study analyses.

These authors also describe the "sample size–phenotype heterogeneity paradox" of data harmonization. That is, although improvements in statistical power are achieved by increasing the sample size using harmonized data, introducing phenotype heterogeneity into the analysis by expanding the sample may alter the ability to detect gene–environment interactions. Similarly, there is a trade-off in that reducing misclassification will improve the validity of G × E analyses, but the cost of collecting rich phenotype data may restrict sample sizes and limit the ranges of environmental variables that can be collected.

## 7.6.2 GEWIS data analysis approaches

The growing interest in GEWIS studies has spurred the development of new statistical methods to characterize gene–environment interactions in the context of genome-wide data. For example, Mukherjee *et al.* (2012) compared the standard case–control approach, the case-only method (Section 7.4), and hybrid methods, including the empirical Bayes and two-stage screening approaches. They showed that, although the case-only method generally provides the most statistical power, it also has the potential to create false-positive tests (inflated type I error), even for large-scale studies in which a small fraction of the genetic markers tested are associated with the exposure being studied. The hybrid methods, however, generally provide an increase in power while controlling type I error. One such method is the empirical Bayes shrinkage method (Mukherjee and Chatterjee, 2008), which is a weighted average of case-only and case–control estimators of interaction. This estimator provides a "tradeoff between bias and efficiency" by weighting the interaction estimator toward the case–control estimator when the assumption of gene–environment independence may be violated, and toward the case-only estimator when this assumption is supported by the data (Mukherjee *et al.*, 2008; Hutter *et al.*, 2012).

Although there is concern about the general validity of the assumption of gene–environment independence, Cornelis *et al.* (2012) examined genome-wide SNP data from two large studies of type 2 diabetes and did not find evidence for inflated type I error using case-only tests. It should be noted, however, that the environmental factor of interest was body mass index, a trait that is also genetically influenced (Thomas *et al.*, 2012). Other authors have described methods that are focused on identifying novel variants that have not been found in searches for marginal genetic effects alone. These include joint tests or two degree of freedom tests of both the gene–environment interaction and the main effect (Kraft *et al.*, 2007; Dai *et al.*, 2012). As another example, Hsu *et al.* (2012) have described "cocktail methods" for detecting genome-wide gene–environment interactions. This approach selects and combines optimal methods from three modules:

1. Module A: Screening steps for prioritizing SNPs using marginal screening, correlation screening, both marginal and correlation screening, or no screening.
2. Module B: Multiple comparison adjustment using Bonferroni corrections, permutation testing, or weighted hypothesis testing.
3. Module C: Gene–environment interaction testing using case–control, case-only, or empirical Bayes testing.

These ongoing developments illustrate that ever more powerful statistical tools are being devised to detect gene–environment interactions exploiting the availability of genome-wide and harmonized environmental data. It should be noted, however, that, since the case-only method is designed to detect interaction only on a multiplicative scale, use of this approach in GEWIS raises the same issues about measurement scale as described in Section 7.3 above.

An analysis of gene–environment interactions and risk of colorectal cancer is illustrated in Box 7.3.

M.A. Austin and R. Ottman

## Box 7.3. Application: Colorectal Cancer (CRC)

As noted in Box 2.2, the heritability of CRC based on data from the Scandinavian twin registries is one of the highest for all cancer sites, 35% (Lichtenstein et al., 2000). Although GWAS have been successful in identifying variants associated with CRC risk, they only explain a small proportion of this heritability, similar to many other complex diseases. Gene–environment interactions may be an important component to CRC risk, and a recent analysis undertook a comprehensive examination of G × E interaction for ten known CRC-associated loci in relation to established environmental risk factors (Hutter et al., 2012).

In order to have sufficient statistical power for such an analysis, large sample sizes are needed, and thus data must be combined across studies. This analysis was based on the Genetic and Epidemiology of Colorectal Cancer Consortium (GECCO) of nine case–control and cohort studies that included 7,016 cases and 9,723 controls. Ten SNPs on nine different chromosomes that had been previously associated with CRC in GWAS were examined, and these are listed in Table 7.9. Among the nine studies, different genotyping platforms had been used, so genotypes for association analyses among the consortium studies were based on imputation using the program BEAGLE with HapMap release 22 as the reference sample (see Chapter 9). Quality control for all genotyping was performed, as were checks for Hardy–Weinberg equilibrium. Of the ten SNPs, eight were associated with CRC risk in the study sample, with nominal p-values ranging from 0.03 to $4.1 \times 10^{-7}$ (Hutter et al., 2012).

The environmental risk factors included in the analysis were body mass index, height, several dietary factors, and aspirin/non-steroidal anti-inflammatory drug use (Table 7.9). Harmonization of these data was a multistep, iterative process, similar to those described in Section 7.6.1, that included:

- identifying common data elements that are "inferentially consistent" by reviewing questionnaires and data dictionaries for each study;
- communicating with each of the participating studies to obtain data and acquire coding information;
- developing standardized variable definitions and consistent coding; and
- transforming data from each study into standardized definitions, and performing quality control, including defining and applying a permissible range of values and logic checks.

The resulting standardized variables were coded as continuous, dichotomous, or ordered categorical variables, or in study-specific quartiles.

To test for gene–environment interactions, the empirical Bayes weighted estimator was used. As described above, this approach provides a weighted average of the case-only and case–control OR. Because a total of 180 interaction tests were performed, with correlation among some of the tests, permutation testing was used to account for multiple comparisons.

Of these 180 tests, six interactions showed nominal p-values <0.01. After adjustment for multiple comparisons, however, only one interaction, rs16892766 SNP (*EIF3H/UTP23*) by vegetable consumption in quartiles, had a p-value <0.05 (permutation-adjusted p = 0.02). Further, there was a dose–response relationship of the effect of the minor allele at rs16892766 by quartile of vegetable consumption: OR = 0.94 for quartile 1, OR = 1.19 for quartile 2, OR = 1.26 for quartile 3, and OR = 1.40 for quartile 4. These results are consistent with an extension of Model E presented in Section 7.2.

*Continued*

**Box 7.3.** Continued.

**Table 7.9.** SNPs and environmental factors considered in gene–environment interaction study of CRC (adapted from Hutter *et al.*, 2012).

| SNP | Chromosomal location | Gene/locus |
|-----|---------------------|------------|
| rs16892766 | 8q23.3 | *EIF3H/UTP23* |
| rs6983267 | 8q24 | *MYC* |
| rs10795668 | 10p14 | *LOC338591* |
| rs3802842 | 11q23 | *LOC120376* |
| rs4444235 | 14q22.2 | *BMP4* |
| rs4779584 | 15q13 | *CRAC1/GREM1* |
| rs9929218 | 16q22.1 | *CDH1* |
| rs4939827 | 18q21 | *SMAD7* |
| rs10411210 | 19q13.1 | *RHPN2* |
| rs961253 | 20p12.3 | *BMP2* |

Environmental factors

Processed meat
Red meat
Body mass index
Smoking
Height
Alcohol consumption
Dietary fiber
Vegetables
Dietary calcium
Fruit
Dietary folate
Aspirin/non-steroidal anti-inflammatory drug use

Taken together, these findings provide evidence for effect modification of rs16892766 SNP (*EIF3H/UTP23*) by vegetable consumption. Elucidating how variants in the region of chromosome 8q23 where this SNP is located may interact with vegetable consumption to alter risk of CRC will be important next steps in this research.

## 7.7 Epistasis: Interactions between Genes

In addition to gene–environment interactions, "Epistasis, or interactions between genes, has long been recognized as fundamentally important to understand the structure and function of genetic pathways ..." (Phillips, 2008). This concept is also central to genetic epidemiology and understanding genetic influences on disease risk.

Similar to the concepts of multiplicative and additive scales of interaction described above, there are also several definitions of epistasis that geneticists have used (Phillips, 1998). In 1909, Bateson originally coined the term epistasis ("standing upon") to describe when one locus masks the effects at another locus, often referred to as functional interaction today. This type of interaction involves molecular interactions between proteins, including when the effects of alleles at one locus are blocked by alleles at another locus, often in the same biological pathway (Phillips, 2008). Using animal models, epistasis then results in a discrepancy between the prediction of segregation ratios based on the action of individual genes, and the actual outcome (phenotype) of a dihybrid cross. The classic example of such interaction is coat color variation in mice. Of the more than 100 loci that control coat color, crosses between *agouti* and melanocortin 1 receptor double-heterozygote mice result in non-Mendelian segregation ratios that have suggested that the melanocortin 1 receptor operates downstream of *agouti*. Crosses with other combinations of mutants have elucidated the biochemistry of this pathway and the proteins involved (Phillips, 2008).

In contrast to this biological definition of interaction between genes, R.A. Fisher (1918) described statistical epistasis (e) as the deviation from the additive combination of two loci in their effects on a phenotype (Phillips, 2008). That is:

$$W_{xy} = a_x + a_y + e$$

where W is phenotype and $a_x$ and $a_y$ are effects of alleles at loci x and y, respectively. Then, in the late 1960s, population geneticists used epistasis as deviation from a multiplicative, rather than an additive, model:

$$W_{xy} = a_x \times a_y + e$$

Hypothesis testing for epistasis using these types of statistical models does not, however, necessarily correspond to biological interactions between proteins (Cordell, 2002). Thus, Phillips (2008) proposes that advances in understanding epistasis and genetic effects that are not predicted from individual components (i.e. main effects) would be facilitated by a "unification" of these biological and statistical views of the concept. This problem is the same as that discussed above in the context of measurement scales for assessment of gene–environment interaction (Madsen *et al.*, 2011b).

Similar to the interest in gene–environment interactions in the context of GWAS described above, it has also been proposed that accounting for epistasis in these studies may improve the detection of genetic influences on complex diseases. That is, an association of a specific variant with disease may not be identified in a GWAS without taking into account its interactions with other genes (Zuk *et al.*, 2012). Cordell (2009) has described a variety of recently developed analysis methods and software to test for interaction between loci. For example, the case-only design can be a powerful approach (see Section 7.4) to test for interactions between known genetic factors, under the assumption that these genotypes are independent in the population. However, because of this assumption, the case-only $\chi^2$ test is not appropriate for closely linked or correlated loci. The empirical Bayes procedure described above, which uses a weighted average of the case-only and case–control estimators, can be also applied in this context. Cordell (2009) emphasizes that the methods being developed, including "exhaustive searches" for all possible two-locus interactions in a GWAS, data-mining methods, and Bayesian model selection approaches, are designed either to test for interactions between loci or to test for association of a specific locus with disease while allowing for interactions.

## 7.8 Conclusion

This chapter has illustrated several approaches to studying interaction in genetic epidemiology, and many challenges remain (Thomas, 2010). Genomic technology is advancing rapidly for characterizing genetic variability, but assessment of exposure continues to involve multidimensional environmental factors and temporal changes that must be refined and harmonized across studies. Large sample sizes are necessary for sufficient power, and improved measures of disease outcome are also needed to reduce heterogeneity and facilitate replication of findings.

Perhaps equally important to these practical challenges, development of a unified conceptual framework that combines statistical scales of interaction with biological views of complex genetic systems would facilitate communication among biologists, geneticists, and epidemiologists, and would be a major advance for genetic epidemiology as well (Institute of Medicine, 2006; Phillips, 2008).

## Acknowledgments

Ruth Ottman was supported by grants from the National Institutes of Health (R01-NS053998, U01-NS07726, U01-NS077367, R01-NS078419). The authors would like to thank Dr Stephen M. Schwartz for providing material in Boxes 7.1 and 7.2, and Dr Carolyn M. Hutter for her careful review of the chapter and for material on GEWIS in Section 7.6.

## Further Reading

Giacomini, K.M., Yee, S.W., Ratain, M.J., Weinshilboum, R.M., Kamatani, N. and Nakamura, Y. (2012) Pharmacogenomics and patient care: one size does not fit all. *Science Translational Medicine* 4, 1–7.

Institute of Medicine (2006) *Gene, Behavior, and the Social Environment. Moving Beyond the Nature/Nuture Debate.* National Academies Press, Washington, DC, pp. 161–180.

Moore, J.H. and Williams, S.M. (2009) Epistasis and its implications for personal genetics. *American Journal of Human Genetics* 85, 309–320.

Thomas, D. (2010) Gene–environment-wide association studies: emerging concepts. *Nature Reviews Genetics* 11, 259–272.

Thomas, D.C., Lewinger, J.P., Murcray, C.E. and Gauderman, W.J. (2012) GE-Whiz! Ratcheting gene–environment studies up to the whole genome and the whole exome. *American Journal of Epidemiology* 175, 203–207.

## References

Albert, P.S., Ratnasinghe, D., Tangrea, J. and Wacholder, S. (2001) Limitations of the case-only design for identifying gene–environment interactions. *American Journal of Epidemiology* 154, 687–693.

M.A. Austin and R. Ottman

Bennett, S.N., Caporaso, N., Fitzpatrick, A.L., Agrawal, A., Barnes, K., Boyd, H.A., *et al.* (2011) Phenotype harmonization and cross-study collaboration in GWAS consortia: the GENEVA experience. *Genetic Epidemiology* 35, 159–173.

Botto, L.D. and Khoury, M.J. (2001) Facing the challenge of gene–environment interaction: the two-by-four table and beyond. *American Journal of Epidemiology* 153, 1016–1020.

Chen, P., Lin, J.J., Lu, C.-S., Ong, C.-T., Hsieh, P.F., Yang, C.-C., *et al.* (2011) Carbamazepine-induced toxic effects and HLA-B*1502 screening in Taiwan. *New England Journal of Medicine* 364,1126–1133.

Chung, W.H., Hung, S.I., Hong, H.S., Hsih, M.S., Yang, L.C., Ho, H.C., *et al.* (2004) Medical genetics: a marker for Stevens–Johnson syndrome. *Nature* 428, 486.

Cordell, H.J. (2002) Epistasis: what it means, what it doesn't mean, and statistical methods to detect it in humans. *Human Molecular Genetics* 11, 2463–2468.

Cordell, H.J. (2009) Detecting gene–gene interactions that underlie human diseases. *Nature Reviews Genetics* 10, 392–404.

Cornelis, M.C., Tchetgen, E.J., Liang, L., Qi, L., Chatterjee, N., Hu, F.B. and Kraft, P. (2012) Gene–environment interactions in genome-wide association studies: a comparative study of tests applied to empirical studies of type 2 diabetes. *American Journal of Epidemiology* 175, 191–202.

Dai, J.Y., Logsdon, B.A., Huang, Y., Hsu, L., Reiner, A.P., Prentice, R.L. and Kooperberg, C. (2012) Simultaneously testing for marginal genetic association and gene–environment interaction. *American Journal of Epidemiology* 176, 164–173.

Fisher, R.A. (1918) The correlation between relatives on the supposition of Mendelian inheritance. *Transactions of the Royal Society of Edinburgh* 52, 399–433.

Fortier, I., Doiron, D., Little, J., Ferretti, V., L'Heureux, F., Stolk, R.P. *et al.* (2011) Is rigorous retrospective harmonization possible? Application of the DataSHaPER approach acorss 53 large studies. *International Journal of Epidemiology* 40, 1314–1328.

Gatto, N.M., Campbell, U.B., Rundle, A.G. and Ahsan, H. (2004) Further development of the case-only study for assessing gene–environment interaction: evaluation of and adjustment for bias. *International Journal of Epidemiology* 33, 1014–1024.

Giacomini, K.M., Yee, S.W., Ratain, M.J., Weinshilboum, R.M., Kamatani, N. and Nakamura, Y. (2012) Pharmacogenomics and patient care: one size does not fit all. *Science Translational Medicine* 4, 1–7.

Greenland, S. and Robins, J.M. (1986) Identifiability, exchangeability, and epidemiological confounding. *International Journal of Epidemiology* 15, 413–419.

Greenland, S. and Robins, J.M. (2009) Identifiability, exchangeability and confounding revisited. *Epidemiology Perspectives and Innovation* 6, 4.

Hamilton, C.M., Strader, L.C., Pratt, J.G., Maiese, D., Hendershot, T., Kwok, R.K. *et al.* (2011) The PhenX Toolkit: get the most from your measures. *American Journal of Epidemiology* 174, 253–260.

Hsu, L., Jiao, S., Dai, J.Y., Hutter, C., Peters, U. and Kooperberg, C. (2012) Powerful cocktail methods for detecting genome-wide gene–environment interaction. *Genetic Epidemiology* 36, 183–194.

Hutter, C.M., Change-Claude, J., Slattery, M.L., Pflugeisen, B.M., Lin, Y., Duggan, D., *et al.* (2012) Characterization of gene–environment interactions for colorectal cancer susceptibility loci. *Cancer Research* 72, 2036–2044.

Institute of Medicine (2006) *Gene, Behavior, and the Social Environment. Moving Beyond the Nature/Nuture Debate.* National Academies Press, Washington, DC, pp. 161–180.

Kasarskis, A.X., Yang, X. and Schadt, E. (2011) Integrative genomics strategies to elucidate the complexity of drug response. *Pharmacogenomics* 12, 1695–1715.

Khoury, M.J. and Flanders, W.D. (1996) Nontraditional epidemiologic approaches in the analysis of gene–environment interaction: case–control studies with no controls! *American Journal of Epidemiology* 144, 207–213.

Khoury, M.J. and Wacholder, S. (2009) From genome-wide association studies to gene–environment-wide interaction studies – challenges and opportunities. *American Journal of Epidemiology* 169, 227–230.

Knol, M.J. and VanderWeele, T.J. (2012) Recommendations for presenting analyses of effect modification and interaction. *International Journal of Epidemiology* 41, 514–520.

Kraft, P., Yen, Y.C., Stram, D.O., Morrison, J. and Gauderman, W.J. (2007) Exploiting gene–environment interaction to detect genetic associations. *Human Heredity* 63, 111–119.

Lichtenstein, P., Holm, N.V., Verkasalo, P.K., Iliadou, A., Kaprio, J., Koskenvuo, M., *et al.* (2000) Environmental and heritable factors in the causation of cancer. *New England Journal of Medicine* 343, 78–85.

Madsen, A.M., Hodge, S.E. and Ottman, R. (2011a) Causal models for investigating complex disease: I. A primer. *Human Heredity* 72, 54–62.

Madsen, A.M., Ottman, R. and Hodge, S.E. (2011b) Causal models for investigating complex genetic disease: II. What causal models can tell us about penetrance for additive, heterogeneity, and multiplicative two-locus models. *Human Heredity* 72, 63–72.

Manolio, T.A., Collins, F.S., Cox, N.J., Goldstein, D.B., Hindorff, L.A., Hunter, D.J., *et al.* (2009) Finding the missing heritability of complex diseases. *Nature* 461, 747–753.

McCormack, M., Alfirevic, A., Bourgeois, S., Farrell, J.J., Kasperaviclute, D., Carrington, M., *et al.* (2011) HLA-A*3101 and carbamazepine-induced hypersensitivity reactions in Europeans. *New England Journal of Medicine* 364, 1134–1143.

Mukherjee, B. and Chatterjee, N. (2008) Exploiting gene–environment independence for analysis of case–control studies: an empirical Bayes-type shrinkage estimator to trade-off between bias and efficiency *Biometrics* 64, 685–694.

Mukherjee, B., Ahn, J., Gruber, S.B., Rennert, G., Moreno, V. and Chatterjee, N. (2008) Tests for gene–environment interaction from case–control data: a novel study of type I error, power and designs. *Genetic Epidemiology* 32, 615–628.

Mukherjee, B., Ahn, J., Gruber, S.B., and Chatterjee, N. (2012) Testing gene–environment interaction in large-scale case–control association studies: possible choices and comparisons. *American Journal of Epidemiology* 175, 177–190.

Ottman, R. (1990) An epidemiologic approach to gene–environment interaction. *Genetic Epidemiology* 7, 177–185.

Ottman, R. (1996) Gene–environment interaction: definitions and study designs. *Preventive Medicine* 25, 764–770.

Phillips, P.C. (1998) The language of gene interaction. *Genetics* 149, 1167–1171.

Phillips, P.C. (2008) Epistasis – the essential role of gene interactions in the structure and evolution of genetic systems. *Nature Reviews Genetics* 9, 855–867.

Psaty, B.M., Smith, N.L., Lemaitre, R.N., Vos, H.I., Heckbert, S.R., LaCroix, A.Z. and Rosendall, F.R. (2001) Hormone replacement therapy, prothrombotic mutation, and the risk of incident nonfatal myocardial infarction in postmenopausal women. *JAMA* 285, 906–913.

Richardson, D.B. and Kaufman, J.S. (2009) Estimation of the relative excess risk due to interaction and associated confidence bounds. *American Journal of Epidemiology* 169, 756–760.

Rothman, K.J. (1976) The estimation of synergy or antagonism. *American Journal of Epidemiology* 103, 506–511.

Rothman, K.J. and Greenland, S. (1998) *Modern Epidemiology*. Lippincott-Raven, Philadelphia, PA.

Thomas, D. (2010) Gene–environment-wide association studies: emerging concepts. *Nature Reviews Genetics* 11, 259–272.

Thomas, D.C., Lewinger, J.P., Murcray, C.E. and Gauderman, W.J. (2012) GE-Whiz! Ratcheting gene–environment studies up to the whole genome and the whole exome. *American Journal of Epidemiology* 175, 203–207.

Umbach, D.M. and Weinberg, C.R. (1997) Designing and analyzing case–control studies to exploit independence of genotype and exposure. *Statistics in Medicine* 16, 1731–1743.

Vandenbroucke, J.P., Koster, T., Briet, E., Reitsma, P.H. Bertina, R.M. and Rosendaal, F.R. (1994) Increased risk of venous thrombosis in oral-contraceptive users who are carriers of factor V Leiden mutation. *Lancet* 344, 1453–1457.

VanderWeele T.J. and Robins J.M. (2007) The identification of synergism in the sufficient-component-cause framework. *Epidemiology* 18, 329–339.

Yang, Q., Khoury, M.J. and Flanders, W.D. (1997) Sample size requirements in case-only study designs to detect gene–environment interaction. *American Journal of Epidemiology* 146,713–720.

Zuk, O., Hechter, E., Sunyaev S.R. and Lander E.S. (2012) The mystery of missing heritability: genetic interactions create phantom heritability. *Proceedings of the National Academy of Sciences USA* 109, 1193–1198.

# 8 Non-Mendelian Genetics

STEPHEN M. SCHWARTZ, PH.D., M.P.H.

*Division of Public Health Sciences Division, Fred Hutchinson Cancer Research Center, and Department of Epidemiology, University of Washington, Seattle, Washington*

## Synopsis

- DNA sequence variation potentially can influence disease risk through mechanisms that do not follow Mendel's laws.
- Non-Mendelian mechanisms include mitochondrial DNA variation, *de novo* variation, and parental and parent-of-origin effects.
- To date, these mechanisms have been primarily examined in either rare conditions or a small subset of common conditions.
- Determining whether non-Mendelian effects account for a measurable proportion of common, complex diseases will require different study designs or additional DNA sources than have been used to identify effects of variants presumably acquired through Mendelian transmission.
- Epigenetic factors – heritable characteristics of chromosomes other than DNA sequence variation that influence gene expression – account for non-Mendelian effects in some rare conditions but their role in common, complex phenotypes is just beginning to be explored.

## 8.1 Introduction

As covered in preceding chapters, the investigation of the contribution of DNA variation to human disease has largely focused on studies, whether of linkage or association, in which the goal is to make inferences about the causative role of variants in the sequence, at one or more base pairs, of an affected individual's nuclear DNA inherited under Mendel's laws. The growing awareness that much of the heritability of complex phenotypes cannot be ascribed to common DNA variation of this type (Eichler *et al.*, 2010) has increased interest in discerning how health is impacted by DNA sequence variation when it is not nuclear in origin, it is not inherited (or expressed) in a Mendelian fashion, or it is carried by a relative but not necessarily the affected individual. In each of these settings, phenotypes among family members would tend to be more similar compared to unrelated individuals (i.e. the traits segregate within families) but the designs and/or analysis approaches described earlier in this book could miss these unconventional relationships between the DNA variation and disease. For reasons that will be explained in the following sections, all of these features prevent researchers from relying on linkage methods for making inferences about the relationship between nucleotide variation and disease, and because linkage methods depend on Mendel's laws, the topics in the chapter are described

© M.A. Austin 2013. *Genetic Epidemiology: Methods and Applications*
(M.A. Austin *et al.*)

broadly as "non-Mendelian genetics". Three types of "non-Mendelian genetics" will be discussed: (i) mitochondrial genome variation; (ii) *de novo* genetic variation; and (iii) parental and parent-of-origin genetic effects. In addition, we summarize the role of epigenetic factors on health, as these probably represent the major mechanism underlying parent-of-origin genetic effects.

## 8.2 Mitochondrial Genetics

Mitochondria are eukaryotic cell structures primarily responsible for the production of stored energy molecules (adenosine triphosphate) through the Krebs cycle and oxidative phosphorylation. Other key roles include cellular calcium homeostasis and mediating apoptotic pathways. Each cell contains thousands of mitochondria, and each mitochondrion contains multiple copies of its own DNA (mtDNA), a double-stranded ~16,500 bp circular molecule consisting of 37 genes (13 encoding proteins necessary for oxidative phosphorylation, 22 encoding tRNA, and two encoding rRNA), and a segment at which replication is initiated (the "D-loop" or control region). Nuclear gene products provide the necessary machinery for mtDNA replication, transcription, translation, and maintenance (Greaves *et al.*, 2012).

Each person's mitochondria originate from the egg of his or her mother, and thus at birth all mtDNA is maternally derived. The uniparental source of mtDNA means that mtDNA variation in health and disease cannot be studied using traditional family designs that capitalize on Mendel's laws. (The same situation applies to studies of variation on the nuclear Y chromosome in men.) It also means that mtDNA variation is more likely than nuclear DNA variation to represent distinct maternal lineages, and hence associations between mtDNA mutations and phenotypes are particularly susceptible to population stratification (see Chapter 6). In addition to mtDNA variation that is maternally inherited, any single mitochondrion can, during life, sustain damage to its DNA resulting in polymorphisms (e.g. single nucleotide polymorphism (SNP), gene deletion) from routine replication error. mtDNA damage becomes established in cells because, in contrast to nuclear DNA, mtDNA is not proofread and consequently does not benefit from repair mechanisms to maintain fidelity. High levels of exposure to DNA-damaging reactive oxygen species can also alter mtDNA variation. And, due to the multiplicity of mitochondria in each cell, any particular tissue from which mtDNA is obtained can contain a mix of mitochondrial genomes consisting of different proportions of any particular mtDNA variant (known as "heteroplasmy"). It is generally believed that acquired mutations need to be present in at least the majority (and in some cases, nearly all) of these organelles for an affected phenotype resulting from an mtDNA variant to be penetrant in a particular tissue. Thus, unlike nuclear DNA variation, which is relatively stable throughout life and identical throughout somatic tissues, the extent and nature of mtDNA variation can be highly dependent on the tissue source and acquired characteristics of the individual. For example, studies have reported that mtDNA variation in buccal cells is related to cigarette smoking (Tan *et al.*, 2008), lymphocyte mtDNA deletions are related to low serum folate (Wu *et al.*, 2009), and the extent of heteroplasmy increases with age (Sondheimer *et al.*, 2011).

## Box 8.1. Application: Breast Cancer

There is strong evidence that oxidative damage to DNA is an important mechanism leading to mutation of proto-oncogenes or tumor suppressor genes, and mitochondria are a major source of reactive oxygen species (Chatterjee *et al.*, 2011). And, one of the hallmarks of cancer is the failure of a cell to respond to apoptotic signals (Hanahan and Weinberg, 2011). Hence, mitochondria are intimately involved in processes that are key to the development of malignancy. Ye *et al.* (2008) hypothesized that women with larger numbers of an mtDNA D-loop region CA repeat polymorphism might be at reduced risk of breast cancer, as prior studies had shown that mitochondrial gene transcription activity is inversely related to CA repeat number, and reduced mitochondrial gene transcription might result in lower levels of oxidative DNA damage (Ye *et al.*, 2008). The authors tested their hypothesis using DNA extracted from blood samples provided by approximately 1,000 cases and 1,000 population-based controls among Chinese women from Shanghai. Relative to women carrying the common $(CA)_5$ and $(CA)_4$ alleles, those carrying at least one copy of the relatively uncommon $(CA)_7$ allele (2.8% allele frequency among controls) were at statistically significantly reduced risk of breast cancer (odds ratio (OR) = 0.50; 95 % confidence interval (CI) = 0.27, 0.93) (Table 8.1). Women who had larger numbers of CA repeats (8–11) were not at reduced risk, however, suggesting that the finding for women with the $(CA)_7$ allele was due to statistical variation. In addition, there was no association between breast cancer risk and whether or not a woman was heteroplasmic for the CA repeat allele. The cases from this study also were followed for 6–8 years for recurrence and survival, and analyses showed that the approximately 10% of the subjects with heteroplasmy (i.e. multiple CA repeat alleles) were at increased risk of death (hazard ratio 1.62; 95% CI = 1.16, 2.26). The authors speculated that heteroplasmy might be a marker of a relatively unstable mitochondrial genome that is prone to mitochondrial dysfunction, which in turn might activate pathways that promote cancer cell survival, and hence, poorer prognosis.

**Table 8.1.** Associations of mtDNA D-loop $(CA)_n$ repeat polymorphism and allele number with breast cancer risk and survival among Chinese women (adapted from Ye *et al.*, 2008).

| Polymorphism | Cases N | Controls N | OR (95% CI) | Cases N | Events[a] N | HR (95% CI) |
|---|---|---|---|---|---|---|
| Genotype | | | | | | |
| $(CA)_5$ | 555 | 587 | 1.0 (reference) | 554 | 160 | 1.0 (reference) |
| $(CA)_4$ | 449 | 468 | 1.02 (0.9, 1.2) | 447 | 115 | 0.86 (0.7, 1.1) |
| $(CA)_6$ | 27 | 34 | 0.84 (0.5, 1.4) | | | |
| $(CA)_7$ | 15 | 32 | 0.50 (0.3, 0.9) | | | |
| $(CA)_{8-11}$ | 12 | 8 | 1.59 (0.6, 3.9) | | | |
| Allele | | | | | | |
| Single allele | 989 | 1013 | 1.0 (reference) | 946 | 250 | 1.0 (reference) |
| Multiple alleles | 109 | 116 | 1.0 (0.8, 1.3) | 109 | 41 | 1.62 (1.2, 2.3) |
| No $(CA)_{6-11}$ allele | 57 | 51 | 1.19 (0.8, 1.8) | 57 | 23 | 1.61 (1.1, 2.5) |
| ≥1 $(CA)_{6-11}$ allele | 52 | 65 | 0.85 (0.6, 1.2) | 52 | 18 | 1.63 (1.0, 2.6) |

[a]Death due to breast cancer or breast cancer recurrence. No associations with survival were estimated for $(CA)_6$, $(CA)_7$, and $(CA)_{8-11}$ genotype carriers due to the small number of cases. HR, hazard ratio.

A number of rare diseases with profound health effects, akin to Mendelian single-gene disorders, have been shown to be due, in whole or in part, to relatively rare mtDNA mutations (Schapira, 2012). For example, mutations within the mitochondrial genes that code for NADH CoQ reductase subunits (11778G→A, 14484T→C, 3460 G→A) cause Leber's hereditary optic neuropathy (Yu-Wai-Man et al., 2011), whereas cases of maternally inherited diabetes and deafness have been reported to be due to a mutation in the mitochondrial tRNA gene MTTL1 (3243A→G) (Yarham et al., 2010). For most "mitochondrial diseases," it is the number of copies of pathogenic mtDNA mutations in the affected tissue that appears to influence disease severity, whereas the extent of circulating mtDNA mutations (i.e. lymphocyte mtDNA as a marker of inherited mtDNA) impacts the chances of transmission from the mother to the next generation. The extent to which lymphocyte mtDNA variation is related to more common, complex phenotypes – particularly those that are known or suspected of having an etiology involving oxidative stress such as cancer and cardiovascular disease (Box 8.1) – has received relatively little study, but somatically acquired mtDNA mutations are of high interest as potential biomarkers of cancer (Chatterjee et al., 2011).

## 8.3   *De Novo* Variation

*De novo* variation refers to the occurrence of nucleotide variation in offspring that is not part of the parent's germ line, i.e. it is "new" to the genome of the family. Nearly all humans have some "small scale" *de novo* variation, with the average individual having 74 new SNPs and three new indels. In contrast, new large copy number variants (CNVs) are much less frequent, occurring in only 2% of individuals (Veltman and Brunner, 2012). The mechanisms by which *de novo* mutations arise, beyond a constant background rate of mutations per nucleotide per generation, are not known. However, several "risk factors" for *de novo* mutations have been identified that may account for its distribution in the population. At the DNA level, *de novo* mutations more commonly occur in regions with greater CpG island density and those affected by segmental duplications (which promote non-allelic homologous recombination). At the person level, individuals with errors in DNA repair capacity or with older fathers are at increased risk of *de novo* mutations. For example, *de novo* point mutations in *FGFR2* increase with increasing paternal age (due to their favorable effect on sperm selection) and are the cause of sporadic conditions such as Apert, Crouzon, and Pfeiffer syndromes (Goriely and Wilkie, 2012). It should be noted that although older fathers are at increased risk of bearing children who have *de novo* mutations (and certain diseases that arise from such mutations), the resulting associations do not technically represent parental or parent-of-origin effects because the risk alleles are not carried by the parent. In general, owing to the absence of evolutionary selection forces, *de novo* mutations are predicted to be much more likely to have profound phenotypic effects than inherited variation (Eyre-Walker and Keightley, 2007). *De novo* mutations can arise in parental gametes, in the embryo, or somatically, and determining which is the source of these variants is an important task not only for understanding the mechanisms of disease development, but for providing information to parents about the risk of recurrence in subsequent offspring (Veltman and Brunner, 2012). For example, if a *de novo* mutation arises in some of a man's spermatogonia, so that some of his sperm carry it but others do not, the sibling recurrence risk could be as high as 50%. In contrast, if the *de novo* mutation occurs in the embryo, it is highly unlikely (given the extremely low background mutation rate per nucleotide) that the family will experience a recurrence of the mutation in a second offspring.

Study designs to identify causative *de novo* mutations require family-based resources but often include samples from unrelated individuals as well (Box 8.2). Family-based samples are typically case–parent trios, in which an initial screen for Mendelian errors (i.e. variants present in the case but not the parents) based on exome sequencing (for detection of SNPs and indels) and/or array comparative genomic hybridization (for detection of large CNVs) provides a set of possible *de novo* mutations. For SNPs and indels, comparisons are then made to sequence data from presumptively unaffected individuals, either related, unrelated, or both, to eliminate previously detected variants. Because high-throughput sequencing in particular is prone to artifacts that can be mistaken for *de novo* mutations (either false positives in offspring or false negatives in parents), extensive additional bioinformatics analyses are employed to eliminate putative hits that could be due to technological limitations of the assays. Finally, Sanger sequencing is used in an attempt to confirm the remaining candidates (Veltman and Brunner, 2012) (see Section 3.6).

---

### Box 8.2. Application: Autism Spectrum Disorders

Autism spectrum disorders (ASDs) are neurodevelopmental conditions marked by a range of language and social interaction impairments (Nazeer and Ghaziuddin, 2012). Although twin studies support the idea that ASDs have a substantial heritable component (Ronald and Hoekstra, 2011), the large proportion of ASDs that appear to be sporadic has prompted the hypothesis that rare, *de novo* DNA variants have a causal role. To test this hypothesis, O'Roak *et al.* sequenced the exomes and detected CNVs in 209 ASD probands and their parents, as well as unaffected siblings of the probands (O'Roak *et al.*, 2012). Predicted *de novo* events in the probands were compared with 2,725 control exomes and those found only in the probands were validated using capillary-based sequencing. Two hundred and forty-eight *de novo* events were identified, and 72% of the probands had at least one non-synonymous *de novo* mutation. Of 51 *de novo* events that could be studied for unambiguous parental origin, 80% occurred on haplotypes inherited from the father, and the number of events per offspring increased with increasing paternal age. The number of *de novo* coding mutations predicted to have severe functional effects per proband was inversely related to non-verbal IQ. The *de novo* mutations identified in this study were found in numerous genes, and although many of the loci were known from prior research to be involved in neurodevelopment, only two of the genes that contained protein-disrupting mutations were affected in more than one proband. Overall, the results support the idea that *de novo* mutations are an important cause of ASDs, and that the loci involved are heterogeneous but tend to belong to well-established biological pathways.

---

S.M. Schwartz

## 8.4 Parental and Parent-of-origin Effects

Parental and parent-of-origin effects pertain to the role that a parent's genetic variation plays in the development of disease in the offspring. With a parental effect, the offspring's disease is related to the DNA variation that one parent carries, regardless of whether or not the offspring has inherited that same variation from the other parent. Such effects are of interest for two reasons. First, the etiology of the offspring's disease may depend on the physiology of a parent, which may be impacted by parental genetic variation. The most obvious candidate phenotypes for maternal genetic effects would be neonatal and childhood conditions (e.g. birth defects, low birth weight, neurodevelopmental disorders, childhood cancers) that have *in utero* origins through the effects, at least in part, of maternal physiology (e.g. Sata *et al.*, 2006; Sharp *et al.*, 2006; Infante-Rivard *et al.*, 2007; Mackelprang *et al.*, 2010; Orjuela *et al.*, 2012; see Box 8.3). Although the idea that a paternal allele which is not inherited can affect offspring disease risk is counter-intuitive (since there is no physical dependence that provides for a father's physiology to affect his son or daughter), the phenomenon has been observed in model organisms but has not yet been explored in humans (Nadeau, 2009; Nelson *et al.*, 2010). Secondly, owing to the fact that each offspring has exactly 50% of each parent's DNA under Mendelian inheritance, the association between an offspring's genotype and his/her disease status is potentially confounded by the association between his/her father or mother's genotype and his/her disease status. That is, if an association exists between paternal genotype and disease, by definition one would observe some association between the offspring genotype and disease that is not due to the offspring carriership of the genotype. Hence, study designs and analytic methods for investigations of offspring genotype effects ideally would account for the possibility of parental genotype effects.

With a parent-of-origin effect, the offspring's disease depends on whether an allele he or she carries was inherited from a particular parent (Guilmatre and Sharp, 2012). Parent-of-origin effects on health first became apparent with the discovery of defects in parent-specific gene expression (known as "imprinting," a type of epigenetic effect: see Section 8.5, below) contributing to rare conditions such as Prader–Willi and Beckwith–Wiedemann syndromes. In Prader–Willi syndrome, for example, the casual "allele" typically is the physical loss of the paternally non-imprinted genes on chromosome 15q11–13 (leaving the imprinted, and thus non-expressed, maternal copies of these genes intact; Butler, 2011). In Beckwith–Wiedemann syndrome, the causal "allele" can occur through loss, or abnormal methylation, of non-imprinted maternal genes (Weksberg *et al.*, 2010). Whether parent-of-origin effects, other than among males due to loci on the X chromosome (which by definition must be due to maternally inherited alleles), play a role in the pathogenesis of common, complex phenotypes has been explored in only a limited number of studies (e.g. Stine *et al.*, 1995; Green *et al.*, 2002; Lindsay *et al.*, 2002; Guo *et al.*, 2006; Bronson *et al.*, 2009; see Box 8.4).

By definition, studies of parental effects and parent-of-origin effects require DNA from both parents in addition to the affected offspring. As with any family-based design, studies of parental effects and parent-of-origin effects are more optimally applied to early-onset conditions than diseases of later life, because this setting increases the chances that the parents will be alive and available to provide specimens.

## Box 8.3. Application: Maternal Genetic Effects and Testicular Germ Cell Tumors

Testicular germ cell tumors (TGCTs) are uncommon in the general population, but are the most common malignancy in young adult men (Sarma *et al.*, 2006). There is extensive evidence that TGCTs are initiated *in utero,* most likely due to a subset of primordial germ cells that, having failed to differentiate into mature germ cells, remains susceptible to the acquisition of oncogenic genetic changes from endogenous or exogenous sources (Rajpert-De Meyts, 2006). The *in utero* origin of TGCTs predicts that a mother's characteristics while pregnant could therefore influence the development of these malignancies. One hypothesized mechanism involves the effect of maternal steroid hormone metabolism on the production of mutation-inducing catechol estrogens. At the same time, the son's steroid hormone metabolism could also influence his risk of TGCT, necessitating a design that can distinguish between maternal and offspring effects. Starr *et al.* therefore studied whether the risk of TGCT would be increased among men whose mothers who carried alleles of cytochrome p450 enzymes predicted to influence the metabolism of steroid hormones, including catechol estrogens (Starr *et al.*, 2005). One hundred and sixty case–parent sets (110 triads and 50 dyads) were genotyped for putatively functional polymorphisms in *CYP1B1* (rs10012, rs1056836, rs1800440), *CYP1A2* (rs762551), *CYP3A4* (rs2740574), and *CYP3A5* (rs776746). The data were analyzed using the log-linear model method developed by Weinberg *et al.* (1998). Notably, maternal carriage of the minor alleles at rs762551 and rs10012 was associated with statistically significant reduced and increased risks, respectively, of TGCT (Table 8.2). In addition, TGCT was strongly associated with offspring (but not maternal) carriership of the rs2740574 minor allele. These results suggest that both a son's and his mother's estrogenic milieu, as represented by nucleotide variation in estrogen-metabolizing genes, influence the son's risk of TGCT.

**Table 8.2.** Relative risk of TGCT associated with maternal and paternal offspring genotypes, by locus (adapted from Starr *et al.*, 2005).

| | Locus | | | | | |
|---|---|---|---|---|---|---|
| | *CYP1A2* | *CYP1B1* | *CYP1B1* | *CYP1B1* | *CYP3A4* | *CYP3A5* |
| | rs762551 | rs10012 | rs1056836 | rs18000440 | rs2740574 | rs776746 |
| | (C/A)[a] | (C/G) | (C/G) | (A/G) | (A/G) | (G/A) |
| Effect | (n = 153)[b] | (n = 150) | (n = 153) | (n = 153) | (n = 158) | (n = 151) |
| **Maternal** | | | | | | |
| MM | 1.0 | 1.0 | 1.0 | 1.0 | 1.0 | 1.0 |
| Mm | 0.4 (0.2, 1.0) | 1.4 (0.8, 2.3) | 0.6 (0.3, 1.1) | 0.9 (0.5, 1.7) | 0.9 (0.4, 2.1) | 0.8 (0.4, 1.5) |
| mm | 0.6 (0.3, 1.5) | 2.6 (1.1, 6.3) | 0.8 (0.4, 1.5) | 0.4 (0.1, 2.1) | 0.9 (0.1, 14) | 0.4 (0.0, 1.2) |
| p[c] | 0.010 | 0.005 | 0.156 | 0.897 | 0.962 | 1.000 |
| **Offspring** | | | | | | |
| MM | 1.0 | 1.0 | 1.0 | 1.0 | 1.0 | 1.0 |
| Mm | 0.7 (0.3, 1.4) | 0.9 (0.5, 1.4) | 1.2 (0.7, 2.0) | 0.8 (0.5, 1.3) | 5.2 (1.5, 1.8) | 1.8 (0.9, 3.6) |
| mm | 0.5 (0.2, 1.2) | 1.0 (0.4, 2.4) | 1.3 (0.6, 2.6) | 0.2 (0.0, 1.4) | ****[d] | **** |
| p | 0.079 | 0.677 | 1.000 | 0.273 | 0.013 | 0.256 |

[a]Major (M) allele /minor (m) allele; [b]numbers in parentheses are number of case–parent triads or dyads; [c]p-values are tests of the hypothesis that the maternal (or offspring) risk allele carriership is associated with offspring TGCT; [d]no offspring were homozygous for the minor allele.

**Box 8.4. Application: Parent-of-origin Effects and Multiple Complex Diseases**

To identify whether published hits from genome-wide association studies (GWAS) (see Section 5.4) of a variety of complex diseases reflected parent-of-origin effects, Kong *et al.* focused on seven validated SNPs for which extensive family data in Iceland were available, and that were near known imprinted genes (Kong *et al.*, 2009). The extensive genealogy database available for Icelanders coupled with novel long-range haplotype phasing permitted assessment of parental genotypes even in the absence of direct genotyping. Five of these SNPs exhibited parent-of-origin specific effects (Table 8.3): rs3817198 (only the paternal T allele associated with breast cancer risk), rs157935 (only the paternal G allele associated with basal cell carcinoma risk), rs231362 (only the maternal T allele associated with type 2 diabetes risk), rs4731702 (the maternal T allele is associated with type 2 diabetes risk), and rs2334499 (the paternal C allele is positively associated with type 2 diabetes risk but the maternal C allele is inversely associated with risk). In a false-discovery rate analysis, the authors estimated that only one of the five parent-of-origin effects that they uncovered was likely to be a spurious finding. These data supported the hypothesis that some common genetic risk factors for complex diseases discovered through GWAS exert their influence through parent-of-origin effects.

**Table 8.3.** Parent-of-origin specific associations with complex diseases in Iceland (adapted from Kong *et al.*, 2009).

| Disease/SNP | Risk allele (MAF) | Paternal OR (p) | Maternal OR (p) | $p^a$ |
|---|---|---|---|---|
| Breast cancer | | | | |
| rs3817198 | T (0.30) | 1.17 (0.038) | 0.91 (0.11) | $6.2 \times 10^{-4}$ |
| Basal cell carcinoma | | | | |
| rs157935 | G (0.68) | 1.40 ($1.5 \times 10^{-6}$) | 1.09 (0.19) | 0.010 |
| Type 2 diabetes | | | | |
| rs2237892 | T (0.93) | 1.03 (0.71) | 1.30 (0.0084) | 0.054 |
| rs231362 | T (0.55) | 0.98 (0.73) | 1.23 ($6.2 \times 10^{-5}$) | 0.0032 |
| rs4731702 | T (0.44) | 0.99 (0.79) | 1.17 (0.001) | 0.022 |
| rs2334499 | C (0.41) | 1.35 ($4.7 \times 10^{-10}$) | 0.86 ($5.7 \times 10^{-11}$) | $4.1 \times 10^{-11}$ |

[a]Test of the difference in frequencies between paternally and maternally inherited risk alleles among cases. MAF, Minor allele frequency; p, p-value.

This limitation no doubt explains the extreme paucity of studies of maternal genetic effects for later-life conditions despite ample evidence for *in utero* effects on diseases of adulthood (Calkins and Devaskar, 2011). Although some studies have attempted to assess parental genetic effects in case–control studies by separately comparing affected offspring (cases) and their parent's genotype frequencies with control genotype frequencies (e.g. van der Put *et al.*, 1995), or the genotypes of parents of cases with genotypes of parents of controls (e.g. Orjuela *et al.*, 2012), these designs do not address the dependence of the parental and offspring genetic effects induced by the Mendelian relationship of genotypes among family members, as discussed above. Thus, these strategies are not capable of assessing whether there are independent maternal, paternal, and/or offspring effects.

The first broadly valid approach developed for estimating independent parental and offspring effects involves genotyping of case–parent trios (see Section 4.2) and a log-linear model analysis based on the counts of trios with different genotype combinations, stratified by the number of copies of the putative risk allele carried by each of the two parents ("parental mating type;" Wilcox et al., 1998). For example, all trios in which the mother carries two risk alleles and the father carries one risk allele, or vice versa, can produce offspring with either one or two risk alleles, and would comprise one parental mating type. In such a design, sometimes it is not possible to recruit both parents for all cases (e.g. if one parent is deceased), but both dyads and triads may be included in these studies by using statistical methods to impute the genotype data for the missing parents (Weinberg, 1999). One limitation of all case–parent trio methods for assessing parental effects is that they essentially are comparing maternal with paternal carriership of the putative risk allele. Thus, a positive association with a maternally carried allele necessarily implies an inverse association with a paternally carried allele, and vice versa. In theory, this limitation could be overcome if the maternal and paternal effects could be estimated independently, as in a hybrid design involving cases, unrelated controls, and mothers and fathers of both cases and controls. In such a design, maternal effects would be assessed by comparing mothers of cases with mothers of controls, and similarly for paternal effects. Another limitation of the case–parent trio approach, as well the case–control/parents of cases and controls approach, is that the parental effects are susceptible to being confounded by population stratification (see Chapter 6). Extending these designs to include grandparents would be needed to address that potential source of bias (Mitchell and Weinberg, 2005), or one could employ one of several techniques to adjust for population stratification statistically (see Chapter 6).

## 8.5  DNA Methylation: An Epigenetic Mechanism Underlying Phenotypic Variation

The epigenome consists of the universe of heritable factors, *aside from DNA sequence*, that influence gene expression, and thus potentially the development of disease as well as other phenotypes (Richards, 2006). Unlike the genome, the architecture of which is extremely well documented due to efforts such as the HapMap and 1000 Genomes projects (International HapMap Consortium, 2003; 1000 Genomes Consortium, 2010), much less is known about the size, scope, organization, and variation of the epigenome. Although substantial progress has recently been made towards characterizing some key components of the epigenome through the NIH Roadmap Epigenomics Mapping Consortium and the ENCyclopedia Of DNA Elements (ENCODE) project (Bernstein *et al.*, 2010, 2012), that the epigenome comprises multiple molecular features (probably including some that have not been discovered) with distinct measurement requirements and tissue specificity continues to pose a great challenge to discerning its scope and role in human health.

The major known types of epigenetic factors are: (i) methylation of cytosines in the DNA sequence (primarily when the cytosine is next to a guanine, i.e. CpG); (ii) chemical modifications of histones (chromosomal proteins that compact DNA

S.M. Schwartz

when it is not being transcribed) including methylation, acetylation, and phosphorylation; and (iii) small RNA molecules contained in germ cells (Richards, 2006). DNA methylation is by far the most extensively characterized epigenetic factor, in part because it has been studied the longest (beginning with the first proposal for its role in gene expression; Holliday and Pugh, 1975), and because assay techniques are based substantially on methods used to analyze nucleotide sequence variation. In humans, DNA methylation affects gene expression by influencing local chromatin structure, with greater amounts of methylation generally leading to reduced affinity for DNA-binding proteins that drive gene transcription. Hence, DNA methylation is generally viewed as a mechanism of silencing genes (as occurs at maternally or paternally imprinted loci (Ferguson-Smith, 2011) or at key tumor suppressor loci in cancers (Estecio and Issa, 2011). DNA methylation, particularly in transposable elements of the genome, is also essential for chromosomal stability.

There are three broad approaches to interrogating a DNA molecule to assess its methylation status, differing primarily in how the DNA samples are prepared for analysis so that it is possible to distinguish methylated and non-methylated DNA (Laird, 2010). The first approach takes advantage of the fact that unmethylated, but not methylated, cytosine can be converted to uracil by treatment with sodium bisulfite. Because uracil pairs with adenine, sodium bisulfite treatment induces a transition polymorphism (cytosine replaced by thymine) at unmethylated loci. The second approach relies on affinity enrichment to isolate methylated DNA sequences using techniques such as immunoprecipitation. The third approach relies on restriction endonucleases that are inhibited by methylated CpG sequences. For each of these approaches, one uses genotyping, sequencing, or arrays to determine the amount and location of methylated DNA at different levels of resolution (ranging from individual base pairs to mega-base-pair regions). For example, genotyping and sequencing of DNA prepared using chemical treatment (bisulfite or restriction endonucleases) can provide single-base-pair resolution, whereas affinity methods provide regional assessments of differential methylation patterns. Affinity methods, however, are cheaper to implement on a genome-wide basis compared with the other approaches. One reasonable strategy that balances the strengths and weaknesses of these approaches begins with affinity-based methods as a discovery step, and then uses chemical treatment methods to target the regions discovered in the discovery step to determine precisely which positions in the DNA sequence are methylated and which are not. Ideally these approaches will eventually be superseded by technologies that measure methylated DNA directly (i.e. without chemical modification or enrichment) as part of DNA sequencing reactions (Flusberg et al., 2010). In addition to these approaches to characterizing the methylation status of specific DNA loci, it is possible to quantify the proportion of cytosines that are methylated throughout a genome using chromatographic and mass spectrometric methods.

The assessment of DNA methylation status, and its relationship to disease risk (Box 8.5), poses multiple challenges compared with corresponding studies of nuclear DNA sequence variation. Most importantly, as with mitochondrial DNA variation (Section 8.2), methylation (and other epigenetic factors) exerts effects in a tissue-specific manner. Thus, while DNA from blood or oral tissue is readily accessible to investigators, methylation patterns in these samples may not reflect tissues in which diseases arise. For example, several studies have reported that methylation levels of blood-derived DNA at CpG positions in *LINE-1* ("long interspersed nucleotide element") are inversely associated with the risk of bladder cancer (Moore *et al.*, 2008; Wilhelm *et al.*, 2010; Cash *et al.*, 2012). *LINE-1* regions are repetitive DNA sequences found throughout the genome that cells normally methylate heavily to avoid chromosomal instability (Estecio and Issa, 2011). The vast majority of DNA methylation occurs in *LINE-1* and related repetitive DNA regions, as opposed to CpG "islands" located near or within specific genes. Investigators subsequently compared *LINE-1* methlyation in peripheral leukocytes, serum, buccal cells and tumor tissue among 50 bladder cancer patients (Van Bemmel, 2012). The proportion of the interrogated CpG positions that were methylated was substantially (and statistically significantly) lower in bladder tumor tissue (61%) than the other sources (range: 77–80%), and there was a poor correlation of *LINE-1* methlyation between bladder tumor and the other tissues (Pearson's correlation coefficients ranged from –0.13 to 0.08). Such results complicate the interpretation of associations between phenotypes and DNA methylation when the latter is measured in "normal" tissue that is not involved in the pathogenesis of the disease. Even within a particular tissue source there can be variation in methylation patterns by cell type (e.g. different immune cells present in peripheral blood (Koestler, 2012)). In addition to tissue heterogeneity, DNA methylation is not static. Studies have shown that DNA methylation is influenced by genetic (Coolen *et al.*, 2011) and environmental factors (Nelson

---

### Box 8.5. Application: Atherosclerosis

Atherosclerosis and its clinical consequences – primarily ischemic heart disease and cerebrovascular disease – are caused in part by low-grade inflammation (Libby, 2012). This response is substantially mediated by peripheral macrophages, which migrate into the arterial wall and serve as a source of cytokines that alter the biology of endothelial and smooth muscle cells towards an atherogenic phenotype (Libby, 2012). Peripheral leukocytes could potentially acquire an atherogenic phenotype through changes in DNA methylation driven by exposure of individuals to cardiovascular risk factors. To determine the relationship between peripheral leukocyte DNA methylation and cardio-vascular disease, investigators conducted a series of analyses within the longitudinal Normative Aging Study of elderly men. Among approximately 700 cohort members alive in 1999 and for whom peripheral leukocyte DNA was collected over the ensuing 8 years, the investigators examined associations between the proportion of methylated cytosines in *LINE-1* repetitive elements and prevalence and incidence of ischemic heart disease and stroke (Baccarreli *et al.*, 2010). *LINE-1* methylation was inversely associated with prevalence of either ischemic heart disease or stroke at baseline, such that men in the lowest quartile (<76% methylation) were at approximately twofold increased risk relative to men in the highest quartile (>79% methylation) (OR = 2.2, 95% CI = 1.2, 3.9). Further, men with *LINE-1* methylation lower than the median (77%) were at threefold increased risk of future ischemic heart disease or stroke (combined) compared with men with methylation levels above the median (HR = 4.1, 95% CI = 1.9, 8.7). These findings were independent of adjustment for cardiovascular disease risk factors, such as age, body mass index, smoking, alcohol consumption, blood pressure, diabetes, serum lipids, and kidney function. These results suggest that genome-wide hypomethylation of peripheral leukocytes is associated with the development of clinical cardiovascular disease, but do not support the idea that the association mediates known risk factors for these conditions.

---

148

S.M. Schwartz

*et al.*, 2011), and decreases with increasing age (Bjornsson *et al.*, 2008; Bollati *et al.*, 2009). Thus, the timing of acquisition of tissues for DNA methylation measurement relative to exogenous exposures as well as the onset of disease is likely to be critical for interpreting associations. For example, methylation patterns in DNA obtained after the disease has manifested itself may reflect the response to physiologic changes brought on by the disease. Such samples could be useful for testing hypotheses about the potential of methylated DNA as an early detection biomarker, but could not be confidently used to draw inferences about the role of methylated DNA as an etiologic factor in the absence of supporting prospectively collected data.

## 8.6 Conclusion

DNA sequence variation potentially can influence disease risk through mechanisms that do not follow Mendel's laws. To date, non-Mendelian mechanisms – mitochondrial DNA variation, parental and parent-of-origin effects, and *de novo* variation – have been primarily examined (and sometimes implicated) in either rare conditions or a small subset of common conditions. Determining whether non-Mendelian effects account for a measurable proportion of common, complex diseases will require different study designs (i.e. based in families rather than unrelated individuals) or additional DNA sources (i.e. affected tissue in addition to peripheral lymphocytes) than have been used in recent years to identify effects of common or rare variants presumably acquired through Mendelian transmission. These same studies would also be well positioned to determine how epigenetic factors contribute to health and, being more amenable to modification than DNA sequence variation, could provide targets for preventive or treatment approaches.

## Acknowledgments

Stephen M. Schwartz was supported by grants and contracts from the US National Institutes of Health (P01CA042792, R01CA095419, R01CA085914, R21ES019709, N01-PC-35142) and by institutional funds from the Fred Hutchinson Cancer Research Center during the writing of this chapter.

## Further Reading

Feinberg, A.P. (2010) Genome-scale approaches to the epigenetics of common human disease. *Virchows Archive* 456, 13–21.

Greaves, L.C., Reeve, A.K., Taylor, R.W. and Turnbull, D.M. (2012) Mitochondrial DNA and disease. *Journal of Pathology* 226, 274–286.

Guilmatre, A. and Sharp, A.J.. (2012) Parent of origin effects. *Clinical Genetics* 81, 201–209.

Labuda, D.A., Krajinovic, M., Sabbagh, A., Infante-Rivard, C. and Sinnett, D. (2002) Parental genotypes in the risk of a complex disease. *American Journal of Human Genetics* 71, 193–197.

Laird, P.W. (2010) Principles and challenges of genomewide DNA methylation analysis. *Nature Reviews Genetics* 11, 191–203.

Nagarajan, R.P., Fouse, S.D. and Costello, J.F. (2013) Methods for cancer epigenome analysis. *Advances in Experimental Medicine and Biology* 754, 313–338.

Richards, E.J. (2006) Inherited epigenetic variation – revisiting soft inheritance. *Nature Reviews Genetics* 7, 395–401.

Satterlee, J.S., Schubeler, D. and Ng, H.H. (2010) Tackling the epigenome: challenges and opportunities for collaboration. *Nature Biotechnology* 28, 1039–1044.

Veltman, J.A. and Brunner, H.G. (2012) *De novo* mutations in human genetic disease. *Nature Reviews Genetics* 13, 565–575.

# References

1000 Genomes Consortium (2010) A map of human genome variation from population-scale sequencing *Nature* 467, 1061–1073.

Baccarelli A., Wright R., Bollati V., Litonjua A., Zanobetti A., Tarantini L., *et al.* (2010) Ischemic heart disease and stroke in relation to blood DNA methylation *Epidemiology* 21, 819–828.

Bernstein, B.E., Stamatoyannopoulos, J.A., Costello, J.F., Ren, B., Milosavljevic, A., Meissner, A., *et al.* (2010) The NIH Roadmap Epigenomics Mapping Consortium. *Nature Biotechnology* 28, 1045–1048.

Bernstein B.E., Birney E., Dunham I., Green E.D., Gunter C. and Snyder M. (2012) An integrated encyclopedia of DNA elements in the human genome. *Nature* 489, 57–74.

Bjornsson, H.T., Sigurdsson, M.I., Fallin, M.D., Irizarry, R.A., Aspelund, T., Cui, H., *et al.* (2008) Intra-individual change over time in DNA methylation with familial clustering. *JAMA* 299, 2877–2883.

Bollati, V., Schwartz, J., Wright, R., Litonjua, A., Tarantini, L., Suh H., *et al.* (2009) Decline in genomic DNA methylation through aging in a cohort of elderly subjects. *Mechanisms of Ageing and Development* 130, 234–239.

Bronson, P.G., Ramsay, P.P., Thomson, G. and Barcellos, L.F. (2009) Analysis of maternal-offspring HLA compatibility, parent-of-origin and non-inherited maternal effects for the classical HLA loci in type 1 diabetes. *Diabetes, Obesity and Metabolism* 11 (Suppl. 1), 74–83.

Butler, M.G. (2011) Prader–Willi Syndrome: obesity due to genomic imprinting. *Current Genomics* 12, 204–215.

Calkins, K. and Devaskar, S.U. (2011) Fetal origins of adult disease. *Current Problems in Pediatric and Adolescent Health Care* 41, 158–176.

Cash H.L., Tao L., Yuan J.M., Marsit C.J., Houseman E.A., Xiang Y.B., *et al.* (2012) *LINE-1* hypomethylation is associated with bladder cancer risk among nonsmoking Chinese. *International Journal of Cancer* 130, 1151–1159.

Chatterjee, A., Dasgupta, S. and Sidransky, D. (2011) Mitochondrial subversion in cancer. *Cancer Prevention Research* 4, 638–654.

Coolen, M.W., Statham, A.L., Qu, W., Campbell, M.J., Henders, A.K., Montgomery, G.W., *et al.* (2011) Impact of the genome on the epigenome is manifested in DNA methylation patterns of imprinted regions in monozygotic and dizygotic twins. *PLoS One* 6, e25590.

Eichler, E.E., Flint, J., Gibson, G., Kong, A., Leal, S.M., Moore, J.H. and Nadeau, J.H. (2010) Missing heritability and strategies for finding the underlying causes of complex disease. *Nature Reviews Genetics* 11, 446–450.

Estecio, M.R. and Issa, J.P. (2011) Dissecting DNA hypermethylation in cancer. *FEBS Letters* 585, 2078–2086.

Eyre-Walker, A. and Keightley, P.D. (2007) The distribution of fitness effects of new mutations. *Nature Reviews Genetics* 8, 610–618.

Ferguson-Smith, A.C. (2011) Genomic imprinting: the emergence of an epigenetic paradigm. *Nature Reviews Genetics* 12, 565–575.

Flusberg, B.A., Webster, D.R., Lee, J.H., Travers, K.J., Olivares, E.C., Clark, T.A., *et al.* (2010) Direct detection of DNA methylation during single-molecule, real-time sequencing. *Nature Methods* 7, 461–465.

Goriely, A. and Wilkie, A.O. (2012) Paternal age effect mutations and selfish spermatogonial selection: causes and consequences for human disease. *American Journal of Human Genetics* 90, 175–200.

Greaves, L.C., Reeve, A.K., Taylor, R.W. and Turnbull, D.M. (2012) Mitochondrial DNA and disease. *Journal of Pathology* 226, 274–286.

Green, J., O'Driscoll, M., Barnes, A., Maher, E.R., Bridge, P., Shields, K. and Parfrey, P.S. (2002) Impact of gender and parent of origin on the phenotypic expression of hereditary nonpolyposis colorectal cancer in a large Newfoundland kindred with a common MSH2 mutation. *Diseases of the Colon & Rectum* 45, 1223–1232.

Guilmatre, A. and Sharp, A.J.. (2012) Parent of origin effects. *Clinical Genetics* 81, 201–209.

Guo, Y.F., Shen, H., Liu, Y.J., Wang, W., Xiong, D.H., Xiao, P., *et al.* (2006) Assessment of genetic linkage and parent-of-origin effects on obesity. *Journal of Clinical Endocrinology & Metabolsim* 91, 4001–4005.

Hanahan, D. and Weinberg, R.A. (2011) Hallmarks of cancer: the next generation. *Cell* 144, 646–674.

Holliday, R. and Pugh, J.E. (1975) DNA modification mechanisms and gene activity during development. *Science* 187, 226–232.

Infante-Rivard, C., Vermunt, J.K. and Weinberg, C.R. (2007) Excess transmission of the NAD(P)H:quinone oxidoreductase 1 (NQO1) C609T polymorphism in families of children with acute lymphoblastic leukemia. *American Journal of Epidemiology* 165, 1248–1254.

International HapMap Consortium (2003) The International HapMap Project. *Nature* 426, 789–796.

Koestler, D.C., Marsit, C.J., Christensen, B.C., Accomando, W., Langevin, S.M., Houseman, E.A., *et al.* (2012) Peripheral blood immune cell methylation profiles are associated with non-hematopoietic cancers. *Cancer Epidemiology Biomarkers and Prevention* 21, 1293–1302.

Kong, A., Steinthorsdottir, V., Masson, G., Thorleifsson, G., Sulem, P., Besenbacher, S., *et al.* (2009) Parental origin of sequence variants associated with complex diseases. *Nature* 462, 868–874.

Laird, P.W. (2010) Principles and challenges of genomewide DNA methylation analysis. *Nature Reviews Genetics* 11, 191–203.

Libby, P. (2012) Inflammation in atherosclerosis. *Arteriosclerosis, Thrombosis and Vascular Biology* 32, 2045–2051.

Lindsay, R.S., Kobes, S., Knowler, W.C. and Hanson, R.L. (2002) Genome-wide linkage analysis assessing parent-of-origin effects in the inheritance of birth weight. *Human Genetics* 110, 503–509.

Mackelprang, R.D., Carrington, M., John-Stewart, G., Lohman-Payne, B., Richardson, B.A., Wamalwa, D., *et al.* (2010) Maternal human leukocyte antigen A*2301 is associated with increased mother-to-child HIV-1 transmission. *Journal of Infectious Diseases* 202, 1273–1277.

Mitchell, L.E. and Weinberg, C.R. (2005) Evaluation of offspring and maternal genetic effects on disease risk using a family-based approach: the "pent" design. *American Journal of Human Genetics* 162, 676–685.

Moore, L.E., Pfeiffer, R.M., Poscablo, C., Real, F.X., Kogevinas, M., Silverman, D., *et al.* (2008) Genomic DNA hypomethylation as a biomarker for bladder cancer susceptibility in the Spanish Bladder Cancer Study: a case–control study. *Lancet Oncology* 9, 359–366.

Nadeau, J.H. (2009) Transgenerational genetic effects on phenotypic variation and disease risk. *Human Molecular Genetics* 18, R202–R210.

Nazeer, A. and Ghaziuddin, M. (2012) Autism spectrum disorders: clinical features and diagnosis. *Pediatric Clinics of North America* 59, 19–25, ix.

Nelson, H.H., Marsit, C.J. and Kelsey K.T. (2011) Global methylation in exposure biology and translational medical science. *Environmental Health Perspectives* 119, 1528–1533.

Nelson, V.R., Spiezio, S.H. and Nadeau, J.H. (2010) Transgenerational genetic effects of the paternal Y chromosome on daughters' phenotypes. *Epigenomics* 2 513–521.

Orjuela, M.A., Cabrera-Munoz, L., Paul, L., Ramirez-Ortiz, M.A., Liu, X., Chen, J., *et al.* (2012) Risk of retinoblastoma is associated with a maternal polymorphism in dihydrofolate-reductase (DHFR) and prenatal folic acid intake. *Cancer* 118, 5912–5919.

O'Roak, B.J., Vives, L., Girirajan, S., Karakoc, E., Krumm, N., Coe, B.P., *et al.* (2012). Sporadic autism exomes reveal a highly interconnected protein network of de novo mutations. *Nature* 485, 246–250.

Rajpert-De Meyts, E. (2006) Developmental model for the pathogenesis of testicular carcinoma in situ: genetic and environmental aspects. *Human Reproduction Update* 12, 303–323.

Richards, E.J. (2006) Inherited epigenetic variation – revisiting soft inheritance. *Nature Reviews Genetics* 7, 395–401.

Ronald, A. and Hoekstra, R.A. (2011) Autism spectrum disorders and autistic traits: a decade of new twin studies. *American Journal of Medical Genetics B Neuropsychiatric Genetics* 156B, 255–274.

Sarma, A.V., McLaughlin, J.C. and Schottenfeld, D. (2006) Testicular cancer. In: Schottenfeld, D. and Fraumeni, J.F. (eds) *Cancer Epidemiology and Prevention*. Oxford University Press, New York, pp. 1151–1165.

Sata, F., Yamada, H., Suzuki, K., Saijo, Y., Yamada, T., Minakami, H. and Kishi, R. (2006) Functional maternal catechol-*O*-methyltransferase polymorphism and fetal growth restriction. *Pharmacogenetics and Genomics* 16, 775–781.

Schapira, A.H. (2012) Mitochondrial diseases. *Lancet* 379, 1825–1834.

Sharp, L., Miedzybrodzka, Z., Cardy, A.H., Inglis, J., Madrigal, L., Barker, S., *et al.* (2006) The C677T polymorphism in the methylenetetrahydrofolate reductase gene (MTHFR), mater-nal use of folic acid supplements, and risk of isolated clubfoot: A case-parent-triad analysis. *American Journal of Epidemiology* 164, 852–861.

Sondheimer, N., Glatz, C.E., Tirone, J.E., Deardorff, M.A., Krieger, A.M. and Hakonarson, H. (2011) Neutral mitochondrial heteroplasmy and the influence of aging. *Human Molecular Genetics* 20, 1653–1659.

Starr, J.R., Chen, C., Doody, D.R., Hsu, L., Ricks, S., Weiss, N.S. and Schwartz, S.M. (2005) Risk of testicular germ cell cancer in relation to variation in maternal and offspring cytochrome p450 genes involved in catechol estrogen metabolism. *Cancer Epidemiology Biomarkers and Prevention* 14, 2183–2190.

Stine, O.C., Xu, J., Koskela, R., McMahon, F.J., Gschwend, M., Friddle, C., *et al.* (1995) Evidence for linkage of bipolar disorder to chromosome 18 with a parent-of-origin effect. *American Journal of Human Genetics* 57, 1384–1394.

Tan, D., Goerlitz, D.S., Dumitrescu, R.G., Han, D., Seillier-Moiseiwitsch, F., Spernak, S.M., *et al.* (2008) Associations between cigarette smoking and mitochondrial DNA abnormalities in buccal cells. *Carcinogenesis* 29, 1170–1177.

Van Bemmel, B.D., Lenz, P., Liao, L.M., Baris, D., Sternberg, L.R., Warner, A., *et al.* (2012) Correlation of *LINE-1* methylation levels in patient-matched buffy coat, serum, buccal cell, and bladder tumor tissue DNA samples. *Cancer Epidemiology Biomarkers and Prevention* 21, 1143–1148.

van der Put, N.M., Steegers-Theunissen, R.P., Frosst, P., Trijbels, F.J., Eskes, T.K., van den Heuvel, L.P., *et al.* (1995) Mutated methylenetetrahydrofolate reductase as a risk factor for spina bifida. *Lancet* 346, 1070–1071.

Veltman, J.A. and Brunner, H.G. (2012) *De novo* mutations in human genetic disease. *Nature Reviews Genetics* 13, 565–575.

Weinberg, C.R. (1999) Allowing for missing parents in genetic studies of case–parents triads. *American Journal of Human Genetics* 64, 1186–1193.

Weinberg, C.R., Wilcox, A.J. and Lie, R.T. (1998) A log-linear approach to case–parent-triad data: assessing effects of disease genes that act either directly or through maternal effects and that may be subject to parental imprinting. *American Journal of Human Genetics* 62, 969–978.

Weksberg, R., Shuman, C. and Beckwith, J.B. (2010) Beckwith–Wiedemann syndrome. *European Journal of Human Genetics* 18, 8–14.

Wilcox, A.J., Weinberg, C.R. and Lie, R.T. (1998) Distinguishing the effects of maternal and offspring genes through studies of "case-parent triads". *American Journal of Epidemiology* 148, 893–901.

Wilhelm, C.S., Kelsey, K.T., Butler, R., Plaza, S., Gagne, L., Zens, M.S., *et al.* (2010) Implications of *LINE1* methylation for bladder cancer risk in women. *Clinical Cancer Research* 16, 1682–1689.

Wu, M.Y., Kuo, C.S., Lin, C.Y., Lu, C.L. and Syu Huang, R.F. (2009) Lymphocytic mitochondrial DNA deletions, biochemical folato status and hepatocellular carcinoma susceptibility in a case–control study. *British Journal of Nutrition* 102, 715–721.

Yarham, J.W., Elson, J.L., Blakely, E.L., McFarland, R. and Taylor, R.W. (2010) Mitochondrial tRNA mutations and disease. *Wiley Interdisciplinary Reviews: RNA* 1, 304–324.

Ye, C., Gao, Y.T., Wen, W., Breyer, J.P., Shu, X.O., Smith, J.R., *et al.* (2008) Association of mitochondrial DNA displacement loop $(CA)_n$ dinucleotide repeat polymorphism with breast cancer risk and survival among Chinese women. *Cancer Epidemiology Biomarkers and Prevention* 17, 2117–2122.

Yu-Wai-Man, P., Griffiths, P.G., Chinnery, P.F. (2011) Mitochondrial optic neuropathies – disease mechanisms and therapeutic strategies. *Progress in Retinal Eye Research* 30, 81–114.

# 9 Software and Data Resources for Genetic Epidemiology Studies

TIMOTHY A. THORNTON, PH.D.

*Department of Biostatistics, University of Washington, Seattle, Washington*

## Synopsis

- Software resources available for genetic epidemiology studies include:
  - R, a free software environment for statistics and graphics;
  - PLINK, a free, open-source software designed to perform a range of analyses;
  - software to account for population structure in genetic association studies, to estimate ancestry, and for genetic relatedness inference;
  - software for power calculations and for imputation of untyped genetic markers; and
  - a comprehensive alphabetical list of genetic analysis software.
- Human reference panels and resources include:
  - HapMap;
  - Human Genetics Diversity Panel (HGDP);
  - 1000 Genomes Project; and
  - Genome Variation Server.
- Genotype and phenotype repositories include:
  - Database of Genotypes and Phenotypes (dbGaP); and
  - European Genome–Phenome Archive (EGA).
- Two examples are presented to illustrate these data and software resources, one characterizing patterns of linkage disequilibrium and another estimating ancestry.

## 9.1 Introduction

Since 1997, tremendous resources have become available for genetic researchers. These include extensive software, genomic databases containing genotype and phenotype data, and population reference panels with high-throughput single nucleotide polymorphism (SNP) genotyping and next-generation sequencing data. Navigating these resources is a challenge that is often encountered in genetic epidemiology studies as there can be difficulty in: (i) identifying and gaining access to suitable genetic data; and (ii) finding appropriate software for the analyses of data. This chapter is designed to aid genetic researchers in identifying resources that are available for genetic epidemiology studies. We will highlight the usefulness of some of these resources and give examples using publicly available genetic data and software.

© M.A. Austin 2013. *Genetic Epidemiology: Methods and Applications* (M.A. Austin *et al.*)

## 9.2 Software for Genetic Data Analysis

### 9.2.1 R software

R (R Development Core Team, 2012) is a free software environment for statistics and graphics. Software packages for the analysis of genetic data are often written in R, and these packages are freely available. As of August 2012, the Comprehensive R Archive Network (CRAN) package repository featured close to 4,000 available packages. Many of these packages are for the analysis of data for genetics and genomics research, and a summary of some of the R packages with statistical methodology and algorithms implemented for the analysis of genetic data can be found on the CRAN website. The R packages available in CRAN are for a broad range of genetic research areas including: population genetics, phylogenetics, linkage, quantitative trait linkage (QTL) mapping, linkage disequilibrium and haplotype mapping, genome-wide association studies (GWAS), and next-generation sequencing.

Another useful resource for the analysis of genetic/genomic data with R is Bioconductor. The Bioconductor project provides a number of R packages for high-throughput genomic data. As of August 2012, the latest release, Bioconductor 2.10, consisted of 554 software packages.

### 9.2.2 PLINK

PLINK (Purcell *et al.*, 2007) is a free, open-source whole-genome association analysis toolset that is widely used by genetic researchers. The software is designed to perform a broad range of large-scale analyses in a computationally efficient manner. PLINK has numerous features for managing and analyzing large genetic data sets. Table 9.1 lists some of the useful tools that have been implemented in PLINK for data management, quality control, and association testing.

### 9.2.3 Software for association testing in samples from structured populations

Chapter 6 gave an overview of a number of the available methods accounting for population structure in genetic association studies. Here we highlight some of the available software packages for the analysis of samples from structured populations.

The EIGENSOFT/EIGENSTRAT software package (Price *et al.*, 2006) is widely used for the analysis of genetic data with population structure in samples with unrelated individuals. This software is capable of performing a principal components analysis (PCA) on large data sets with millions of markers. In samples of unrelated individuals with population structure, the top principal components can reflect ancestry differences among the sample individuals, and the EIGENSTRAT method implemented in this software package can be used to perform valid genetic association testing in the presence of population structure, where the top principal components are used as covariates in a linear regression model to adjust for population structure.

**Table 9.1.** PLINK tools for data management, quality control, and association testing.

| PLINK usage | Implemented features and tools |
| --- | --- |
| Data management | Reads data in a variety of formats |
| | Allows for recoding and reordering of alleles in files |
| | Multiple files with genetic data can be merged into a single file |
| | Subsets (SNPs or individuals) can be extracted and printed to a file |
| | Allows for the flipping of DNA strands for SNPs (useful feature when merging data sets genotyped on different arrays/platforms is required) |
| Quality control | Can perform Hardy–Weinberg equilibrium tests and also provides both allele and genotype frequencies for SNPs |
| | Provides missing genotype rates |
| | Inbreeding, identical-by-state (IBS) and identical-by-descent (IBD) statistics for individuals and pairs of individuals |
| | Identifies non-Mendelian transmission of alleles in family data |
| | Sex checks based on X chromosome SNPs |
| | Tests of non-random genotyping failure |
| Association testing | Case–control association tests (see Purcell *et al.*, 2007) include: (i) standard allelic test; (ii) Cochran–Armitage trend test; (iii) Mantel–Haenszel and Breslow–Day tests for stratified samples; (iv) tests for dominant/recessive, additive, multiplicative, and general disease models; and (v) model comparisons tests (e.g. general disease model versus additive) |
| | Family-based association (transmission disequilibrium test (TDT), sibship tests) |
| | Quantitative trait association |
| | Association testing conditional on multiple SNPs |
| | Allows for both assessment of significance based on asymptotic and/or empirical p-values |
| | SNP "set-based" or "gene-based" association tests (see Purcell *et al.*, 2007) |
| | Detecting epistasis (interaction of SNPs that influence a trait; see Chapter 7) |
| | Tests for gene–environment interaction with continuous and dichotomous environments |

For association testing in samples with both population structure and relatedness, the ROADTRIPS (Thornton and McPeek, 2010) and EMMAX (Kang *et al.*, 2010) software packages can be used. The ROADTRIPS software is for case–control study designs, whereas EMMAX is for studies with quantitative traits but can also allow for dichotomous traits.

### 9.2.4 Individual ancestry estimation software

The STRUCTURE software (Pritchard *et al.*, 2000) can be used for estimating proportional ancestry with a small number of ancestry informative genetic markers. STRUCTURE uses a Bayesian approach based on a Markov chain Monte Carlo (MCMC) algorithm for simultaneously estimating individual ancestry proportions and ancestral allele frequencies at the markers.

T.A. Thornton

For estimating individual ancestry and ancestral allele frequencies, the ADMIXTURE software (Alexander *et al.*, 2009) incorporates a similar likelihood model to that implemented in STRUCTURE but with an improved algorithm so that the method is computationally feasible for large-scale GWAS. ADMIXTURE runs significantly faster than STRUCTURE where analyses can be completed in minutes with ADMIXTURE that can take hours with STRUCTURE. An example of an application with the ADMIXTURE software for individual ancestry estimation of a Mexican American sample is given in Box 9.1. The FRAPPE software package (Tang *et al.*, 2005) can also be used to estimate individual ancestry in large-scale genetic data. FRAPPE implements an expectation–maximization (EM) algorithm for simultaneously inferring each individual's ancestry proportion and allele frequencies in the ancestral populations. In our applications of the FRAPPE and ADMIXTURE software to samples with ancestry admixture, we have found that the two software packages give nearly identical individual ancestry estimates.

---

**Box 9.1. Examples using Publicly Available Genetic Data and Software Resources**

**Patterns of linkage disequilibrium in the HapMap YRI and CEU**

The Haploview software (Barrett *et al.*, 2005) can be used for graphical displays of LD in a sample. Haploview software takes as input a SNP genotype data file for sample individuals and then displays as output the LD patterns for the sample in a chromosomal region of interest. Plate 6a and 6b are plots of the LD patterns obtained using Haploview for the HapMap YRI and CEU, respectively, for a 200 kb region on chromosome 2. In these figures, bright red represents high LD, shades of pink show less LD, and blue shows low LD. As one can see, the LD pattern in this region on chromosome 22 is different for the two populations, which illustrates that LD patterns are often population specific. In particular, the areas of high LD, outlined in black, differ considerably for the two groups.

**Ancestry estimation in the HapMap Mexican Americans (MXL)**

We used publicly available reference panels and software for estimating individual ancestry in the HapMap Mexican Americans in the Los Angeles, California (MXL) population. This HapMap MXL sample consists of 86 individuals. To estimate ancestry in the HapMap MXL, the ADMIXTURE software was used, where the HapMap CEU and YRI samples were used as surrogates for African and European ancestry, respectively, and the HGDP Native American samples (NAM) were used as surrogates for Native American ancestry. The HGDP and HapMap samples were genotyped on different arrays/platforms, so the PLINK software was used to: (i) combine the HapMap and HGDP samples into a single file; (ii) flip strands of DNA at SNPs that were discordant so that strands were the same for the two platforms; and (iii) create a genotype date file for the ADMIXTURE software including only the HapMap and HGDP samples needed for the analysis as well as the SNPs genotyped on both platforms.

*Continued*

---

**Box 9.1.** Continued.

Plate 7 presents a bar plot, created using the R software, of the results from an ADMIXTURE analysis of the HapMap MXL sample in which the HGDP NAM and HapMap CEU and YRI samples were included in the analysis as fixed groups (green, blue, and red, respectively), and proportional ancestry was estimated for the 86 HapMap MXL genotyped individuals (Y axis). In the bar plot of the ADMIXTURE ancestry estimates, the HapMAP MXL individuals are arranged in increasing order (left to right) of genome-wide Native American ancestry proportion. All HapMap MXL individuals have modest African ancestry, around 5% on average with a standard deviation of 0.02; most of their ancestry is European and Native American at around 50% and 45%, respectively, on average. The proportion of European and Native American ancestry is quite variable, with the Native American ancestry proportion ranging from 0.04 to 0.81 and having a standard deviation of 0.15, and the European ancestry proportion ranging from 0.18 to 0.93 and also having a standard deviation of 0.15. HapMap MXL individual ancestry estimates were recently used to identify cryptic relatedness in the sample with the REAP method (Thornton *et al.*, 2012).

## 9.2.5  Relatedness estimation software for GWAS

Identity-by-descent (IBD) sharing probabilities and kinship coefficients are commonly used measures of genetic relatedness. Alleles at a genetic locus that are inherited copies of a common ancestral allele are said to be IBD. (The term IBD is generally used to refer to recent, as opposed to ancient, common ancestry.) Pairs of non-inbred individuals (i.e. individuals with unrelated parents) can share 0, 1, or 2 alleles IBD. The kinship coefficient for a pair of individuals is defined to be the probability that a random allele selected from the first individual in the pair and a random allele selected from second individual in the pair at a locus are IBD. The kinship coefficient for a non-inbred pair can be written as a function of the IBD sharing probabilities, where the kinship coefficient is equal to $1/2 \times$ P(sharing 2 alleles IBD) + $1/4 \times$ P(sharing 1 allele IBD). Table 9.2 gives IBD sharing probabilities and kinship coefficients for relative pairs.

**Table 9.2.** Expected kinship coefficients and IBD sharing probabilities for non-inbred relationships.

| Relationship | Kinship coefficient | Probability of IBD = 0 | Probability of IBD = 1 | Probability of IBD = 2 |
|---|---|---|---|---|
| Monozygotic twins | 0.5 | 0 | 0 | 1 |
| Parent–offspring | 0.25 | 0 | 1 | 0 |
| Full siblings | 0.25 | 0.25 | 0.5 | 0.25 |
| Second-degree | 0.125 | 0.5 | 0.5 | 0 |
| Third-degree | 0.0625 | 0.75 | 0.25 | 0 |
| Fourth-degree | 0.03125 | 0.875 | 0.125 | 0 |
| Unrelated pairs | 0 | 1 | 0 | 0 |

T.A. Thornton

A problem often encountered in GWAS is that of identifying cryptic relatedness in a sample, because it is well known that inclusion of genetically related individuals can invalidate association test statistics if not properly addressed either by removing related individuals from the analysis or by adjusting for them in the analysis stage (Kang *et al.*, 2010; Thornton and McPeek, 2010). For inferring relatedness in GWAS samples derived from a single, homogenous population, the previously mentioned PLINK software can be used. PLINK implements a method of moments (MOM) algorithm for estimating IBD sharing probabilities and kinship coefficients based on genome-screen data and SNP allele frequencies that are calculated from the sample. The relatedness estimators implemented in PLINK work well in relatively homogenous samples but have been shown to give biased relatedness estimates in the presence of population structure.

For relatedness inference in structured samples from ancestrally distinct subpopulations, the KING (kinship-based inference for GWAS)-robust method (Manichaikul *et al.*, 2010) can be used for estimating kinship coefficients. In lieu of using sample-level allele frequencies when estimating kinship coefficients for pairs of individuals, an approach that leads to biased estimates in the presence of population structure, KING-robust estimates kinship coefficients by using shared genotype counts as a measure of genetic distance between individuals.

A number of populations, such as African Americans and Hispanics, have population structure due to ancestral admixture of chromosomes from different continents, and simplified population structure assumptions such as population homogeneity and ancestrally distinct samples do not hold. For estimating relatedness in structured populations with admixed ancestry, the REAP (relatedness estimation in admixed populations) method (Thornton *et al.*, 2012) can be used. REAP provides robust estimation of IBD sharing probabilities and kinship coefficients in admixed populations by appropriately accounting for population structure and ancestry-related assortative mating by using individual-specific allele frequencies at SNPs that are calculated on the basis of ancestry derived from whole-genome analysis.

### 9.2.6 Software for power calculations in genetic association studies

Study design plays a critical role in the success (or failure) of a genetic epidemiology study. An essential first step in the planning of a genetic study of this type is to determine the number of samples required to achieve sufficient power to detect plausible genetic effects for a trait of interest. A power analysis is also useful after conducting a genetic epidemiology study. For example, for a study with no significant findings, determining the smallest detectable effect size based on the size of the study sample can be useful for gaining insight as to whether or not the study was underpowered. Fortunately, there are software packages available for calculating: (i) power for a given study design for a fixed number of samples; and (ii) the number of sample individuals that will be needed for a study to have a desired level of power for different effect sizes. The Quanto software can be used for computing both sample size and power for association studies of genes, gene–environment interaction, and gene–gene interaction. The program allows for a variety of study designs including both matched and unmatched case–control, case–sibling, case–parent, and case-only designs. Quanto can also calculate power for quantitative traits.

The Genetic Power Calculator (GPC) software (Purcell *et al.*, 2003) is a useful program for power calculations of variance components methods for both linkage and association mapping. GPC can calculate power for sibships of arbitrary size, where the user inputs levels of the proportion of variance explained by a trait locus that is acting additively and/or has a dominance component. The software also provides power calculations for testing association for dichotomous traits with the transmission disequilibrium test for trio-based study designs (where there are two parents and one affected offspring), as well power for a case–control design.

### 9.2.7   Genotype imputation software

Genotype imputation is often used to infer genotypes at untyped markers in GWAS. Most genotype imputation algorithms match genotype data at typed SNPs in sample individuals to haplotypes from suitable reference panels, and then predict or impute genotypes that are not directly assayed in the sample based on the markers in the reference haplotypes. Genotype imputation can be used in GWAS to test untyped genetic markers for association, as well as to combine results of genome-wide association scans that are genotyped on different platforms. There are a number of available genotype imputation methods that have been implemented in software for GWAS, including IMPUTE (Howie *et al.*, 2009), MACH (Li *et al.*, 2010), fastPHASE (Scheet and Stephens, 2006), and BEAGLE (Browning and Browning, 2009). A detailed description and comparison of these and other imputation methods can be found in a recent review paper (Marchini and Howie, 2010).

### 9.2.8   An alphabetical list of genetic analysis software

A useful resource for identifying software that may be useful for the analysis of genetic data is a website containing a list of software in alphabetical order (Alphabetical List of Genetic Analysis Software). This website contains descriptions of hundreds of available software packages for the analysis of genetic data and URL links for downloading the software packages. Software for a broad spectrum of genetic research areas can be found on this website including: population genetics, genetic linkage analysis for human pedigree data, QTL analysis for animal/plant breeding data, genetic marker ordering, genetic association analysis, haplotype construction, and pedigree drawing. One of the widely used software programs for the analysis of haplotypes and LD block structures listed on this website is Haploview (Barrett *et al.*, 2005). An application of the Haploview software with SNP genotype data from European and African ancestry samples can be found in Box 9.1. Most of the software packages listed are freely available, but some software must be purchased to use.

## 9.3   Human Reference Panels and Resources

### 9.3.1   International Haplotype Map Project (HapMap)

The International Haplotype Map Project (International HapMap 3 Consortium, 2010) began in 2002 with a goal of cataloging common human genetic variation across several populations. The project has had three phases. Phases I and II of HapMap provided high-throughput genotyping SNP data for 3 million SNPs in a sample consisting of 270 individuals from four populations: Yoruba in Ibadan, Nigeria (YRI); Japanese in Tokyo, Japan (JPT); Han Chinese in Beijing, China (CHB); and Utah residents with ancestry from Northern and Western Europe (CEU). Phase III of HapMap includes samples from the original four populations that were represented in phases I and II as well as samples from the following seven additional populations: Luhya in Webuye, Kenya (LWK); Maasai in Kinyawa, Kenya (MKK); Toscani in Italy (TSI); Gujarati Indians in Houston, Texas (GIH); Chinese in Metropolitan Denver, Colorado (CHD); Mexican Americans in Los Angeles, California (MXL); and African Americans from the south-western USA (ASW). The latest HapMap release, release 3 of phase III, contains genotype data for close to 1.5 million SNPs across the genome for 1,397 individuals from the 11 populations.

## 9.3.2 1000 Genomes Project

The 1000 Genomes Project started in 2008 with a goal of finding most genetic variants that have frequencies of at least 1% in samples from various populations via genome sequencing. The latest phase of the project, Phase 2, consists of low coverage and exome next-generation sequencing data (with approximately 36 million SNPs, 4 million indels, and 14,000 deletions) for sample individuals from 19 populations. A list of the 19 different populations represented in Phase 2 of the 1000 Genomes Project can be found in Table 9.3.

**Table 9.3.** Population samples in the 1000 Genomes Project.

| Population | Population abbreviation |
| --- | --- |
| African Caribbean in Barbados | ACB |
| HapMap African ancestry individuals from SW USA | ASW |
| Chinese Dai in Xishuangbanna, China | CDX |
| Center for the Study of Human Polymorphisms (CEPH) individuals | CEU |
| Han Chinese in Beijing | CHB |
| Chinese in metropolitan Denver, Colorado | CHD |
| Han Chinese South | CHS |
| Colombian in Medellin, Colombia | CLM |
| HapMap Finnish individuals from Finland | FIN |
| British individuals from England and Scotland | GBR |
| HapMap Gujarati India individuals from Texas | GIH |
| Iberian populations in Spain | IBS |
| Japanese individuals | JPT |
| Kinh in Ho Chi Minh City, Vietnam | KHV |
| Luhya individuals | LWK |
| HapMap Maasai individuals from Kenya | MKK |
| HapMap Mexican individuals from Los Angeles, California | MXL |
| Peruvian in Lima, Peru | PEL |
| Puerto Rican in Puerto Rico | PUR |

Note that 11 of the 19 population samples given in Table 9.3 that were sequenced in the 1000 Genomes Project are the 11 sample populations from the HapMap project.

### 9.3.3 Human Genetic Diversity Panel (HGDP)

The Human Genetic Diversity Panel (HGDP) (Li *et al.*, 2008) was started by a group of scientists at Stanford University who collaborated on a large study to understand genetic diversity in human populations. In this study, 1,064 individuals from 52 populations were sampled from around the world (Cavalli-Sforza, 2005) and were genotyped on the Illumina 650Y array, a high-throughput genotyping array containing more than 650K SNPS across the genome. Table 9.4 lists the 52 populations that are represented in the HGDP reference panel by geographic regions.

### 9.3.4 Genome Variation Server

The Genome Variation Server (GVS) is local database hosted by the SeattleSNPs Program for Genomic Applications (PGA). GVS contains a database of genomic

**Table 9.4.** Populations represented in the HGDP

| Geographic region | Population | Geographic region | Population |
|---|---|---|---|
| Europe | Orcadian | Eastern Asia | Xibo |
| | Adyegi | | Yi |
| | Russian | | Mongola |
| | Basque | | Naxi |
| | French | | Cambodian |
| | North Italian | | Japanese |
| | Sardinia | | Yakut |
| | Tuscan | Central and Southern Asia | Balochi |
| Africa | Bantu | | Brahui |
| | Mandenka | | Makrani |
| | Yoruba | | Sindhi |
| | San | | Pathan |
| | Mbuti pygmy | | Burusho |
| | Blaka | | Hazara |
| | Mozabite | | Uygur |
| Eastern Asia | Han (S. China) | | Kalash |
| | Han (N. China) | Western Asia | Bedouin |
| | Dai | | Druze |
| | Daur | | Palestinian |
| | Hezhen | Oceania | Melanesian |
| | Lahu | | Papuan |
| | Miao | Americas | Karitiana |
| | Oroqen | | Surui |
| | She | | Colombian |
| | Tujia | | Maya |
| | Tu | | Pima |

T.A. Thornton

data for a number of reference population samples, including the samples from HapMap and the 1000 Genomes Project, and provides rapid access to this data as well as tools to analyze genotype data in the database. Some of the useful feature of GVS include allowing the user to specify a list of genes, chromosome regions, or SNPs for a population of interest for printing genotypes, SNP summary information, linkage disequilibrium (LD) values, tag SNPs, or haplotypes to files.

## 9.4  Genotype and Phenotype Repositories

The database of Genotypes and Phenotypes (dbGaP) was developed to archive and distribute the results of studies that have investigated genotypes and phenotypes. Studies that are available include: GWAS, medical sequencing studies, and molecular diagnostic assays, as well as studies of association between genotype and non-clinical traits. Some of the data are publicly available data, whereas other data are controlled-access data, where researchers must apply to gain access. A recent exploratory analysis of 2,724 data access requests approved between June 2007 and August 2010 found that dbGaP has facilitated secondary research for investigators from academic, governmental, and non-profit and for-profit institutions in the USA and abroad (Walker *et al.*, 2011).

The European Genome–Phenome Archive (EGA) is a repository containing genotype and phenotype information for a number of genetic studies conducted in Europe. EGA is the repository that holds the well-known Wellcome Trust Case Control Consortium genotype and phenotype data.

## 9.5  Conclusion

This chapter has highlighted a variety of currently available resources for genetic epidemiology research. Software resources include: R, a free software environment for statistics and graphics; PLINK, a free, open-source software designed to perform a range of analyses; software to account for population structure in genetic association studies, to estimate ancestry, and for genetic relatedness inference; and software for power calculations and for imputation of untyped genetic markers, as well as a comprehensive alphabetical list of genetic analysis software. Human reference panels include HapMap, the 1000 Genomes Project, the Genome Variation Server, and the database of Genotypes and Phenotypes. Two examples illustrating the use of these data and software resources, one for LD and one for ancestry estimation, have been presented.

## Acknowledgments

Preparation of this chapter was supported in part by the National Institutes of Health grant K01 CA148958. The content is solely the responsibility of the author and does not necessarily represent the official views of the National Institutes of Health.

# Further Reading

Elston, R.C., Satagopan, J.M. and Sun, S. (2012) *Statistical Human Genetics: Methods and Protocols*. Humana Press, New York.

Gogarten, S.M., Bhangale, T., Conomos, M.P., Laurie, C.A., McHugh, C.P., Painter, I., *et al.* (2012) GWASTools: an R/Bioconductor package for quality control and analysis of genome-wide association studies. *Bioinformatics* 28, 3329–3331.

Price, A.L., Zaitlen, N.A., Reich, D. and Patterson N. (2010) New approaches to population stratification in genome-wide association studies. *Nature Reviews Genetics* 11, 459–463.

Seldin, M., Pasaniuc, B. and Price, A. (2011) New approaches to disease mapping in admixed populations. *Nature Reviews Genetics* 12, 523–528.

# References

Alexander, D.H., Novembre, J. and Lange, K. (2009) Fast model-based estimation of ancestry in unrelated individuals. *Genome Research* 19, 1655–1664.

Barrett, J.C., Fry, B., Maller, J. and Daly, M.J. (2005) Haploview: analysis and visualization of LD and haplotype maps. *Bioinformatics* 21, 263–265.

Browning, B. and Browning, S. (2009) A unified approach to genotype imputation and haplotype-phase inference for large data sets of trios and unrelated individuals. *American Journal of Human Genetics* 84, 210–223.

Cavalli-Sforza, L.L. (2005) The Human Genome Diversity Project: past, present and future. *Nature Reviews Genetics* 6, 333–340.

Howie, B.N., Donnelly, P. and Marchini, J. (2009) A flexible and accurate genotype imputation method for the next generation of genome-wide association studies. *PLoS Genetics* 5, e1000529.

International HapMap 3 Consortium (2010) Integrating common and rare genetic variation in diverse human populations. *Nature* 467, 52–58.

Kang, H.M., Sul, J.H., Zaitlen, N.A., Kong, S., Freimer, N.B., Sabatti, C. and Eskin, E. (2010) Variance component model to account for sample structure in genome-wide association studies. *Nature Genetics* 42, 348–354.

Li, J.Z., Absher, D.M., Tang, H., Southwick, A.M., Casto, A.M., Ramachandran, S., *et al.* (2008) Worldwide human relationships inferred from genome-wide patterns of variation. *Science* 319, 1100–1104.

Li, Y., Willer, C.J., Ding, J., Scheet, P. and Abecasis, G.R. (2010) MaCH: using sequence and genotype data to estimate haplotypes and unobserved genotypes. *Genetic Epidemiology* 34, 816–834.

Manichaikul, A., Mychaleckyj, J.C., Rich, S.S., Daly, K., Sale, M. and Chen, W.M. (2010) Robust relationship inference in genome-wide association studies. *Bioinformatics* 26, 2867–2873.

Marchini, J. and Howie, B. (2010) Genotype imputation for genome-wide association studies. *Nature Reviews Genetics* 11, 499–511.

Price, A.L., Patterson, N.J., Plenge, R.M., Weinblatt, M.E., Shadick, N.A. and Reich, D. (2006) Principal components analysis corrects for stratification in genome-wide association studies. *Nature Genetics* 38, 904–909.

Pritchard, J.K., Stephens, M. and Donnelly, P. (2000) Inference of population structure using multilocus genotype data. *Genetics* 155, 945–959.

Purcell, S., Cherny, S.S. and Sham, P.C. (2003) Genetic Power Calculator: design of linkage and association genetic mapping studies of complex traits. *Bioinformatics* 19, 149–150.

T.A. Thornton

Purcell, S., Neale, B., Todd-Brown, K., Thomas, L., Ferreira, M.A.R., Bender D., *et al.* (2007). PLINK: a toolset for whole-genome association and population-based linkage analysis. *American Journal of Human Genetics* 81, 559–575.

R Development Core Team (2012) *R: a Language and Environment for Statistical Computing.* R Foundation for Statistical Computing, Vienna, Austria.

Scheet, P. and Stephens, M. (2006) A fast and flexible statistical model for large-scale population genotype data: applications to inferring missing genotypes and haplotypic phase. *American Journal of Human Genetics* 78, 629–644.

Tang, H., Peng, J., Wang, P. and Risch, N.J. (2005) Estimation of individual admixture: analytical and study design considerations. *Genetic Epidemiology* 28, 289–301.

Thornton, T. and McPeek, M.S. (2010) ROADTRIPS: case–control association testing with partially or completely unknown population and pedigree structure. *American Journal of Human Genetics* 86, 172–184.

Thornton, T., Tang, H., Hoffmann, T.J., Ochs-Balcom, H.M., Caan, B.J. and Risch, N. (2012) Estimating kinship in admixed populations. *American Journal of Human Genetics* 91, 122–138.

Walker, L., Starks, H., West, K.M. and Fullerton, S.M. (2011) dbGaP data access requests: a call for greater transparency. *Science Translational Medicine* 3, 113cm34.

# Web Resources

All web resources accessed on September 21, 2012.

1000 Genomes Project data available at: http://www.1000genomes.org

ADMIXTURE software available at: https://www.genetics.ucla.edu/software/admixture/index.html

Alphabetical List of Genetic Analysis software available at: http://linkage.rockefeller.edu/soft/

BEAGLE software available at: http://faculty.washington.edu/browning/beagle/beagle.html

Bioconducter website available at: http://www.bioconductor.org/

CRAN website available at: http://cran.r-project.org/web/views/Genetics.html

Database of Genotypes and Phenotypes (dbGaP) repository available at: http://www.ncbi.nlm.nih.gov/gap

EIGENSOFT/EIGENSTRAT software available at: http://genepath.med.harvard.edu/~reich/Software.htm

EMMAX software available at: http://genetics.cs.ucla.edu/emmax/

European Genome-Phenome Archive (EGA) repository available at: http://www.ebi.ac.uk/ega/

fastPHASE software available at: http://stephenslab.uchicago.edu/software.html

FRAPPE software available at: http://med.stanford.edu/tanglab/software/frappe.html

Genome Variation Server (GVS) available at: http://gvs.gs.washington.edu/GVS/index.jsp

Genetic Power Calculator (GPC) software available at http://pngu.mgh.harvard.edu/~purcell/gpc/

Haploview software available at: http://www.broad.mit.edu/mpg/haploview/

Human Genetic Diversity Panel (HGDP) data available at: http://hagsc.org/hgdp/index.html

IMPUTE software available at: https://mathgen.stats.ox.ac.uk/impute/impute.html

International HapMap Consortium (HapMap) data available at: http://hapmap.ncbi.nlm.nih.gov/

KING software available at: http://people.virginia.edu/~wc9c/KING/

MACH software available at: http://www.sph.umich.edu/csg/abecasis/MACH

PLINK software available at: http://pngu.mgh.harvard.edu/~purcell/plink/

Quanto software available at http://hydra.usc.edu/GxE

R software available at: http://www.R-project.org/

REAP software available at: http://faculty.washington.edu/tathornt/software/index.html

ROADTRIPS software available at: http://galton.uchicago.edu/~mcpeek/software/index.html

STRUCTURE software available at http://pritch.bsd.uchicago.edu/software.html

# 10 Ethical Issues in Genetic Epidemiology

STEPHANIE M. FULLERTON, D.PHIL.
AND KELLY EDWARDS, PH.D.

*Department of Bioethics and Humanities, University of Washington, Seattle, Washington*

## Synopsis

- Genetic epidemiology studies require the voluntary participation of patients and healthy individuals, whose genomic and phenotypic data are essential for advancing scientific discovery.
- All research involving living human subjects is guided by a set of federal regulations known as "the Common Rule" that are based on three core ethical principles: Respect for Persons, Beneficence, and Justice.
- Respect for Persons is operationalized as informed consent to participate in research. Ideally, participants should understand the nature of the study, the likely risks, benefits, and uncertainties, and that their participation is voluntary.
- Participants may value having an ongoing say in research decision making, especially where future uses of data and specimens are difficult to predict at the time of initial recruitment.
- Elements of research governance for a genetic epidemiology study include participant recruitment, data storage and management, consent, data access, return of results to participants, communication, and oversight.

## 10.1 Introduction

Genetic epidemiology and other forms of human genetic research require the voluntary participation of patients and healthy individuals, whose genomic and linked phenotypic data are essential for advancing scientific discovery. Such researcher–participant interactions pose a host of important regulatory and ethical concerns that should be addressed at the earliest stages of designing and implementing a given program of research.

## 10.2 Current Regulatory Environment

All research involving living human subjects (hereafter "participants") is guided by a set of federal regulations referred to collectively as "the Common Rule" because the policy applies to activities overseen by 17 different federal agencies (US Department of Health and Human Services, 2009). These regulations, which are based in

© M.A. Austin 2013. *Genetic Epidemiology: Methods and Applications*
(M.A. Austin *et al.*)

recommendations of the Belmont Report (Belmont Report, 1979), outline require-ments for the conduct of research including obtaining and documenting informed consent, as well as institutional oversight of research and compliance with applicable laws. Belmont emphasized three core ethical principles as relevant to the conduct and review of human subjects research:

- *Respect for Persons*: protecting the autonomy of all people and treating them with courtesy and respect.
- *Beneficence*: maximizing good outcomes for humanity and research subjects, while minimizing or avoiding risks or harm.
- *Justice*: ensuring reasonable, non-exploitative, and well-considered procedures are administered fairly (the fair distribution of costs and benefits).

The impetus for these ethical principles, and subsequent regulations, was a legacy of abuse within research, where people were subjected to treatments or exposed to disease without their permission or, in some cases, without their knowl-edge (e.g. Beecher, 1966). For many genetic epidemiologists, this backdrop feels quite disconnected from the nature of the research performed in current genetic epidemiology studies today. Indeed, in most genetic epidemiological research there are no direct physical risks beyond a blood draw, and even fewer in the case of secondary analyses of existing data or blood. Instead, the primary risks to partici-pants are more often regarded as risks to privacy, with the confidentiality of genetic and linked phenotypic (including clinical) information being a key locus of regula-tory concern. One straightforward way to attend to concerns about participant privacy is to de-identify samples and linked data so that the contributing individual can no longer be readily identified.

Accordingly, and since 2004, the Office of Human Research Protections (OHRP) has modified their regulations to exempt research using information or specimens derived from living, but otherwise de-identified, participants from human subjects oversight (Office of Human Research Protections, 2008). In other words, it has been determined that any remaining risks to participants are effectively mitigated by removing identifying information. This allows secondary investigators, i.e. those who use data to ask and answer questions but do not interact directly with partici-pants, to pursue their investigations without obtaining additional consent or the sign off of an Institutional Review Board (IRB). Although this guidance seems to be responsive to the original conception of risk as based in threats to individual privacy, and has been effective in expediting research review, in practice, there are a number of limitations:

- It is now accepted that genetic information is itself an identifier (McGuire and Gibbs, 2006).
- The focus on individual risks to identity ignores potential harms to groups (McGregor, 2007).
- State laws trump Federal ones, which leads to complexity, particularly in multi-site studies or where data collected in one jurisdiction must be submitted to fed-eral data repositories.
- There are examples of participants objecting to uses of their data and specimens about which they were not informed, e.g. research uses of blood spots collected from newborns for public health screening purposes (Roser, 2010).

The regulatory guidance on the oversight of de-identified data and specimens has been sufficiently controversial that changes have recently been proposed. Specifically, in a suggested Revision to the Common Rule announced in 2011 (Office of Human Research Protections, 2011) regulators have proposed requiring informed consent for all biospecimen research, regardless of de-identification. Others, such as the Presidential Commission for the Study of Bioethical Issues (Presidential Commission, 2012), have also been actively soliciting comment on the oversight of genomic research. The current regulatory environment is therefore likely to change in the near future (Emanuel and Menikoff, 2011).

## 10.3  Trade-offs of Data De-identification

As noted above, de-identification as the preferred remedy for mitigating informational risks to participants is complicated by the fact that, in most genetic epidemiological research, even modest amounts of genetic information render a sample theoretically identifiable (McGuire and Gibbs, 2006). Although a genetic profile is not nearly as readily identifying as a name, address, or social security number, it is true that, if there is an identified sample against which to compare, the systematic consideration of a surprising small number of unlinked genetic loci (15–25) can result in the identification of a participant's data. Indeed, it is the fundamentally unique nature of any given individual's genetic profile that forms the basis of forensic genetic approaches now used routinely in law enforcement. More unexpected was the subsequent demonstration that, where larger numbers of genetic markers are in play (e.g. a genome-wide association study), individual research participants can even be readily identified from *aggregate* genotypic information, i.e. where genotypes are pooled across potentially hundreds of cases or controls (Homer *et al.*, 2008). Together, these observations have led bioethicists and other privacy experts to question whether it is right to promise participants that their data can be protected in this way (Fullerton *et al.*, 2010; Ohm, 2010).

Leaving aside the question of whether de-identification is feasible as a matter of practice, a number of additional considerations suggest that scientists would be wise to think carefully before choosing to work exclusively with de-identified data. First, although many genetic epidemiological analyses are cross-sectional by design, there will also be instances in which having the ability to go back to specific research participants, either to collect additional data for longitudinal analyses and disease incidence, or to enlist the involvement of biological relatives, may be necessary and/or desirable. If participants' data have been de-identified, such re-contact becomes impossible, rendering the participants' individual contributions to research less valuable than they might otherwise have been. In other words, following the ethical principle of non-maleficence or minimizing harm might significantly, albeit inadvertently, interfere with the maximization of research benefit.

A second important trade-off involves the ability to re-contact participants when individual findings of special health significance are uncovered in the course of research. Although the return of individual genetic research findings has been extensively debated (Bredenoord *et al.*, 2011), there is an emerging consensus

S.M. Fullerton and K. Edwards

(Fabsitz *et al.*, 2010) that researchers should offer individual findings in a timely manner where the following conditions are met:

- A genetic finding has important health implications and the associated risks are established and substantial.
- There are established therapeutic or preventative interventions or other available actions that have the potential to change the clinical course of disease.
- The test is analytically valid and the disclosure plan complies with all applicable laws.
- During the informed consent process or subsequently, the study participant has opted to receive his or her individual results.

Obviously, de-identification effectively precludes such return and may place researchers in the untenable position of knowing clinically valuable (and, in rare instances, urgent) information but being unable to convey what they know to the affected participant. Nor is it sufficient to conclude that one's research activities are not likely to generate clinically actionable information. Potentially returnable findings may be identified incidentally in a variety of ways, including routine data quality checks that stumble across sex chromosomal anomalies and other clinically actionable genotypes (Fullerton *et al.*, 2012). With widespread adoption of whole-exome and whole-genome sequencing approaches in genetic epidemiological research the incidental identification of clinically important information will become even more likely.

These trade-offs must be weighed carefully against the potential harms of re-identification, including the possibility that information about genetic predispositions may be used in harmful ways, e.g. in employment or insurance discrimination. The Genetic Information Non-Discrimination Act or GINA, passed by the US Congress in 2008, prohibits genetic discrimination in employment and health insurance underwriting, but does not extend its protections to life or long-term care insurance (Department of Health and Human Services, 2009). Although the likelihood of having one's genetic information misused is currently low, it is genuinely difficult to predict how such risks may change as genetic testing in both direct-to-consumer and clinical contexts becomes more pervasive.

## 10.4 Informed Consent and Respect

Despite important trade-offs, de-identification remains the preferred way of protecting participants' data and, as noted above, current regulations allow secondary research use of de-identified data in the absence of ongoing oversight or consent. Nevertheless, most participants in genetic epidemiological research do provide informed consent at the time that they are initially recruited, whether to a specific study or a standing biorepository. There is a longstanding legal and ethical tradition which suggests, as a matter of respect for persons, that individuals consent to participate in research. Ideally, this consent should be fully informed, meaning participants should understand the nature of the study, the likely risks, benefits, and uncertainties, and that their participation is voluntary (Faden and Beauchamp, 1986). Participants should also understand how their information will be protected, who will have access to their identifiable data, whether or not individual results will be returned, and what will happen to their data if they later decide to withdraw from the study. Having such information to hand in advance of agreeing to participate allows individuals to make a free and informed decision about contributing their personal information to research.

While the desirability of informed consent at study recruitment is unambiguous, and certain elements of consent documentation are proscribed as a matter of research regulation (Code of Federal Regulations, 2005), in practice investigators (and their institutions) have latitude with regard to how they approach the consent process and identify, or constrain, individual participants' preferences with respect to their research participation. For instance, different research groups are using a range of approaches when collecting and using data in genetic epidemiological research, such as:

- notifying patients of possible specimen or data use in research and providing an "opt-out" option;
- asking participants to give "broad" (i.e. open-ended) consent for unspecified future uses;
- giving "tiered" consent options, where participants can specify their preferences regarding issues such as re-contact, limiting the nature of research (e.g. to cancer studies, or health studies only), and/or restricting use to one institution or research group;
- re-contacting for re-consent at each novel research use; and
- consenting to a process or governance structure that would make clear how future research decisions and decisions about a need to re-contact participants would be made.

Which approach to informed consent is the "best" and in what regard (i.e. most aligned with participant preferences, fair, or transparent) is actively debated. This debate is taking place against the background of several recent high-profile cases, in which research participants (or others involved in unconsented research using de-identified data) have sued researchers for giving misleading (Harmon, 2010) or non-existent (Roser, 2010) informed consent. These cases have highlighted public concerns about research practices that, though legally permissible and in many cases routine, may also be regarded as disrespectful of participant and/or community values. For some, the fundamental trustworthiness of biomedical research, including genetic epidemiological research, is called into question by such examples.

The role that informed consent can or should play in the research process can be complex, as illustrated in experiences with one recent project. Researchers at the Group Health Research Institute in Seattle became involved in a national research consortium called the Electronic Medical Records and Genomics (eMERGE) network (McCarty et al., 2011). For that collaboration, they agreed to make available to other investigators in the consortia genetic and clinical data associated with a longitudinal prospective cohort investigation focused on dementia, and to place de-identified copies of the data in the federal data repository dbGaP (Database of Genotypes and Phenotypes) (Mailman et al., 2007). However, although the informed consent documentation for the cohort study described plans to share data with outside collaborators, there was no language to suggest that sharing would be as extensive as allowed by dbGaP deposition. The IRB therefore asked investigators to return to research participants to seek additional consent (re-consent) for dbGaP-related data sharing.

S.M. Fullerton and K. Edwards

Studies at four other sites in the consortium, with roughly equivalent consent language, decided that additional permission was not required before data were shared via the repository (McGuire *et al.*, 2011).

Re-consent was sought from 1,340 study participants; 86% of these (1,159) agreed to dbGaP deposition, and 365 of those who re-consented were subsequently surveyed by telephone (Ludman *et al.*, 2010). Despite the high rate of re-consent, a majority of survey respondents reported that it was very (69%) or somewhat (21%) important that they had been asked for their permission to have data shared with the federal repository. In addition, many respondents considered alternatives to consent, such as notification-only or opt-out, to be unacceptable (67% and 40%, respectively), whereas 70% suggested that it would have been unacceptable if their data had been shared with neither notification or permission. Cohort participants appreciated being given a say, not because wide sharing was inherently objectionable but because the request represented a demonstration of researchers' trustworthiness and regard (Trinidad *et al.*, 2011).

## 10.5 Research Governance

Studies like the one conducted at Group Health suggest that research participants may value having a greater say in research decision making, especially where future uses of data and specimens are difficult to predict at the time of initial recruitment. Various online tools are emerging to facilitate a more dynamic approach to re-contact and information sharing (Kaye *et al.*, 2012a). In most current cases, however, it is infeasible to re-approach participants for permission for each new collaboration or previously unanticipated research use. This has led to renewed interest in identifying research governance mechanisms that might stand in for more elaborate consent processes and enhance accountability and trustworthiness while promoting effective use of hard-to-come-by participant data.

The term "governance" can be used in various ways. In the broadest sense, governance is a "multifaceted compound situation of institutions, systems, structures, processes, procedures, practices, relationships and leadership behavior in the exercise of social, political, economic, and managerial/administrative authority in the running of public or private affairs" (Kaye *et al.*, 2012b). In biomedical research, governance typically means giving attention to decision-making processes and structures throughout the course of specimen or data collection, handling, distribution, and use. Greater reliance on governance also means that potential participants are asked not to agree to a defined research protocol (led by identified collaborators for specific research purposes) but rather to agree to a set of principles relating to the ways in which research may be conducted, overseen by a group entrusted to represent the interests of participants (Kaye *et al.*, 2012b). The advantage of such an approach is that it allows investigators to respond flexibly, and reasonably quickly, to changing research circumstances – such as the availability of new methods – while doing so in a way that is attentive to participants' values and perspectives. Governance should therefore be adaptive and responsive to local context. In the best cases, the governance mechanisms will be informed more directly by participant voices either through membership on decision-making boards or through consultation with advisory committees (O'Doherty *et al.*, 2011).

**Table 10.1.** Elements of research governance to address at the earliest stages of research.

| Element | Relevant questions |
|---|---|
| Purpose | • What is the goal of the research collection? |
| Recruitment | • Study eligibility? |
| | • Timing and context of approach? |
| Data storage and management | • Where and how will data be stored? |
| Consent | • What kind of consent will be used? |
| Data access | • How will data access requests be reviewed? By whom? |
| | • Who is eligible to make requests? |
| | • For what kinds of purposes? |
| | • What data use agreement requirements? |
| Return of results | • To participants? |
| | • To repository? |
| Communication | • Will uses and outcomes of the research collection be shared with others (public, participants, researchers)? |
| | • What modalities will be used? How often will updates be made? |
| Oversight | • By whom and how? |
| | • Will participant representatives be consulted or included in the governance? |
| | • How often will governance processes be audited or reviewed? |

Research studies can vary considerably with regard to the form of governance ultimately adopted, depending on size, purpose, population, and local history. Regardless of those variables, there are a number of elements every researcher or collection director will need to make about a collection of data or specimens (Table 10.1). In a larger collection, there may be different committees appointed to set policy and review individual decisions in each category, whereas in a smaller collection, a single investigator may serve all functions him- or herself.

Several different metaphors are in use to describe the management of research collections, from owner (perhaps the most familiar to an individual researcher who has established his or her own collection), to custodian, to steward. Circumstances will dictate the appropriate framework for the research collection. In any case, transparency and ongoing communication or availability of information about processes and products will facilitate trustworthy research practices (Yarborough *et al.*, 2009).

## 10.6 Conclusion

Genetic epidemiology and other forms of human genetic research require the voluntary participation of patients and healthy individuals, whose genomic and linked phenotypic data are essential for advancing scientific discovery. Current regulations governing human subjects research favor risk mitigation,

S.M. Fullerton and K. Edwards

operationalized as data de-identification, over other forms of respectful engagement. Nevertheless, varied evidence suggests that participants may value having a greater say in research decision making, especially where future uses of data and specimens are difficult to predict at the time of initial recruitment. New adaptive approaches to research governance may provide a more effective way of maximizing secondary uses of specimens and data while respecting participants' altruistic contributions to research.

## Acknowledgments

The authors acknowledge the support of the University of Washington (UW) Center for Genomics and Healthcare Equality (NHGRI P50 HG3374, W. Burke, PI), the UW Center for Ecogenetics & Environmental Health (NIEHS P30 ES07033, D. Eaton, PI), and the Institute for Translational Health Sciences (NCRR UL1 RR025014, M.L. Disis, PI), as well as the UW Institute for Public Health Genetics.

## Further Reading

Belmont Report (1979) The Belmont Report: ethical principles and guidelines for the protection of human subjects of research. Available from: http://www.hhs.gov/ohrp/humansubjects/guidance/belmont.html (accessed August 21, 2012).

Bredenoord, A.L., Kroes, H.Y., Cuppen, E., Parker, M. and van Delden, J.J. (2011) Disclosure of individual genetic data to research participants: the debate reconsidered. *Trends in Genetics* 27, 41–47.

O'Doherty, K.C., Burgess, M.M., Edwards, K., Gallagher, R.P., Hawkins, A.K., Kaye, J., *et al.* (2011) From consent to institutions: designing adaptive governance for genomic biobanks. *Social Science and Medicine* 73, 367–374.

## References

Beecher, H.K. (1966) Ethics and clinical research. *New England Journal of Medicine*, 274, 1354–1360.

Belmont Report (1979) The Belmont Report: ethical principles and guidelines for the protection of human subjects of research. Available from: http://www.hhs.gov/ohrp/humansubjects/guidance/belmont.html (accessed August 21, 2012).

Bredenoord, A.L., Kroes, H.Y., Cuppen, E., Parker, M. and van Delden, J.J. (2011) Disclosure of individual genetic data to research participants: the debate reconsidered. *Trends in Genetics,* 27, 41–47.

Code of Federal Regulations (2005) Title 45: Public welfare, Part 46 – Protection of human subjects, Subpart A – Basic HHS Policy of protection of human research subjects. Section 116, General requirements for informed consent. Available from: http://ecfr.gpoaccess.gov/cgi/t/text/text-idx?c=ecfr&sid=7abd6573a877027d6ca86f53d966ac44&rgn=div8&view=text&node=45:1.0.1.1.25.1.1.14&idno=45 (accessed August 21, 2012).

Department of Health and Human Services (2009) "GINA" The Genetic Information Nondiscrimination Act of 2008: information for researchers and health care professionals. Available from: http://www.genome.gov/Pages/PolicyEthics/GeneticDiscrimination/GINAInfoDoc.pdf (accessed August 21, 2012).

Emanuel, E.J. and Menikoff, J. (2011) Reforming the regulations governing research with human subjects. *New England Journal of Medicine*, 365, 1145–1150.

Fabsitz, R.R., McGuire, A., Sharp, R.R., Puggal, M., Beskow, L.M., Biesecker, L.G., *et al.* (2010) Ethical and practical guidelines for reporting genetic research results to study participants: updated guidelines from a National Heart, Lung, and Blood Institute working group. *Circulation Cardiovascular Genetics* 3, 547–590.

Faden, R.R. and Beauchamp, T.L. (1986) *A History and Theory of Informed Consent*. Oxford University Press, New York.

Fullerton, S.M., Anderson, N.R., Guzauskas, G., Freeman, D. and Fryer-Edwards, K. (2010) Meeting the governance challenges of next-generation biorepository research. *Science Translational Medicine* 2, 15cm13.

Fullerton, S.M., Wolf, W.A., Brothers, K.B., Clayton, E.W., Crawford, D.C., Denny, J.C., *et al.* (2012) Return of individual research results from genome-wide association studies: experience of the Electronic Medical Records and Genomics (eMERGE) network. *Genetics in Medicine* 14, 424–431.

Harmon, A. (2010) Havasupai case highlights risks in DNA research. *New York Times*, April 21.

Homer, N., Szelinger, S., Redman, M., Duggan, D., Tembe, W., Pearson, J.V., *et al.* (2008) Resolving individuals contributing trace amounts of DNA to highly complex mixture using high-density SNP genotyping microarrays. *PLoS Genetics* 4, e1000665.

Kaye, J., Curren, L., Anderson, N., Edwards, K., Fullerton, S.M., Kanellopoulou, N., *et al.* (2012a) From patients to partners: participant-centric initiatives in biomedical research. *Nature Reviews Genetics* 13, 371–376.

Kaye, J., Gibbons, S.M., Heeney, C., Parker, M. and Smart, A. (2012b) *Governing Biobanks – Understanding the Interplay between Law and Practice*. Hart Publishing, Oxford, UK.

Ludman, E.J., Fullerton, S.M., Spangler, L., Trinidad, S. B., Fujii, M.M., Jarvik, G.P., *et al.* (2010) Glad you asked: participants' opinions of re-consent for dbGap data submission. *Journal of Empirical Research on Human Research Ethics* 5, 9–16.

Mailman, M. D., Feolo, M., Jin, Y., Kimura, M., Tryka, K., Bagoutdinov, R., *et al.* (2007) The NCBI dbGaP database of genotypes and phenotypes. *Nature Genetics* 39, 1181–1186.

McCarty, C.A. Chisholm, R.L., Chute, C.G., Kullo, I.J., Jarvik, G.P., Larson, E.B., *et al.* (2011) The eMERGE Network: a consortium of biorepositories linked to electronic medical records data for conducting genomic studies. *BMC Medical Genomics* 4, 13.

McGregor, J.L. (2007) Population genomics and research ethics with socially identifiable groups. *Journal of Law, Medicine and Ethics* 35, 356–370.

McGuire, A.L. and Gibbs, R.A. (2006) No longer de-identified. *Science* 312, 370–371.

McGuire, A.L., Basford, M., Dressler, L.G., Fullerton, S.M., Koenig, B.A., Li, R., *et al.* (2011) Ethical and practical challenges of sharing data from genome-wide association studies: the eMERGE Consortium experience. *Genome Research* 21, 1001–1007.

O'Doherty, K.C., Burgess, M.M., Edwards, K., Gallagher, R.P., Hawkins, A.K., Kaye, J., *et al.* (2011) From consent to institutions: designing adaptive governance for genomic biobanks. *Social Science and Medicine* 73, 367–374.

Office of Human Research Protections (2008) Guidance on research involving coded private information or biological specimens. Available from: http://www.hhs.gov/ohrp/policy/cdebiol.html (accessed August 21, 2012).

Office of Human Research Protections (2011) Information related to Advanced Notice of Proposed Rulemaking (ANPRM) for Revisions to the Common Rule. Available from: http://www.hhs.gov/ohrp/humansubjects/anprm2011page.html (accessed August 21, 2012).

Ohm, P. (2010) Broken promises of privacy: responding to the surprising failure of anonymization. *UCLA Law Review* 57, 1701.

Presidential Commission (2012) Obama's bioethics commission to meet in D.C. May 9, 2012. Available from: http://bioethics.gov/cms/node/684 (accessed August 21, 2012).

Roser, M.A. (2010) State illegally traded, sold newborns' blood to private companies, suit alleges: Texas Civil Rights Project claims health department deceived public. *Austin American-Stateman*, December 8.

Trinidad, S.B., Fullerton S.M., Ludman, E.J., Jarvik G.P., Larson, E.B. and Burke, W. (2011) Research practice and participant preferences: the growing gulf. *Science* 331, 287–288.

US Department of Health and Human Services (2009) Code of Federal Regulations: Title 45 Public Welfare, Part 46 Protection of Human Subjects. Available at: http://www.hhs.gov/ohrp/humansubjects/guidance/45cfr46.html/ (accessed August 21, 2012).

Yarborough, M., Fryer-Edwards, K., Geller, G. and Sharp, R. (2009) Transforming the culture of biomedical research from compliance to trustworthiness: insights from non-medical sectors. *Academic Medicine* 84, 472–477.

# 11 Public Health and Clinical Applications of Genetic Epidemiology

MARTA GWINN, M.D., M.P.H.[1]
AND W. DAVID DOTSON, PH.D.[2]

[1]McKing Consulting Corporation, Office of Public Health Genomics, Centers for Disease Control and Prevention, Atlanta, Georgia; [2]Office of Public Health Genomics, Centers for Disease Control and Prevention, Atlanta, Georgia

## Synopsis

- Public health has an interest in ensuring that proposed applications of genomic research are scientifically valid and that they add value to existing practice and programs.
- As the basic science of public health, epidemiology contributes key concepts and approaches to translation, which we describe in four phases:
  - T1: Discovery to candidate health application.
  - T2: Health application to evidence-based guidelines.
  - T3: Guidelines to health practice.
  - T4: Practice to population health impact.
- Each of these phases is illustrated using cascade screening for Lynch syndrome as an example.
- Translating genetic epidemiology research presents new opportunities to bridge clinical medicine with public health.

## 11.1 Introduction

> Molecular biology, especially once the human genome is mapped,
> must surely turn increasingly to the study of populations.
> (Kerr L. White, 1991)

At the start of the Human Genome Project, Kerr White – a founder of the field of health services research – suggested that epidemiologists would have a key role in using genetic information to define individual and collective health risks. He hoped that this endeavor would help "heal the schism" that divides medicine from public health in many countries, especially the USA (White, 1991). In fact, several developments of the last decade have encouraged new connections between laboratory-based, basic bio-medical sciences and population-based, public health research. The rise of genetic association studies has introduced molecular scientists to epidemiologic methods (Cordell and Clayton, 2005). Better access to genomic technologies and data has given genetic epidemiologists new tools for measurement and analysis (Thomas, 2000).

© M.A. Austin 2013. *Genetic Epidemiology: Methods and Applications*
(M.A. Austin *et al.*)

The fast-paced flurry of gene discoveries that followed completion of the Human Genome Project fed expectations that health benefits would soon follow; however, the translation of genome research into applications for medicine and public health remains slow and uncertain. In this respect, genomics is much like other biomedical research; for example, a frequently cited analysis found that the average publication interval between a promising discovery and a relevant clinical trial was more than 16 years (Contopoulos-Ioannidis et al., 2008). Moreover, this step from "bench to bedside" constitutes only the first stage in translation from research to practice and public health outcomes.

Public health genomics can be defined as "the responsible and effective translation of genome-based knowledge for the benefit of population health" (Burke et al., 2006; Khoury et al., 2007). In this chapter, we use a framework summarized briefly in Table 11.1 to describe the vital role of epidemiology in each of four phases of translation. Subsequent sections of this chapter describe each phase in more detail, using cascade screening for Lynch syndrome as an example. The last column of Table 11.1 contains references relevant to the Lynch syndrome example.

## 11.2 T1: From Discovery to Candidate Health Application

A full understanding of disease will require capturing much of
the genetic variation across the human population.
(Eric D. Green, 2011)

Today, genomics and other "omics" sciences are threaded throughout the biomedical enterprise. Between 2000 and 2011, the National Library of Medicine's PubMed

Table 11.1. The role of epidemiology at each phase of translating human genomics research (adapted from Khoury et al., 2010a), with examples related to cascade screening for Lynch syndrome.

| | Translation phase | Epidemiologic research approaches | Example (references): cascade screening for Lynch syndrome |
|---|---|---|---|
| T1 | Discovery to candidate health application | Family studies<br>Case–control and cohort studies<br>Phase I and II clinical trials | (Lynch et al., 1966)<br>(Watson and Lynch, 2001; Giráldez et al., 2012) |
| T2 | Health application to evidence-based guidelines | Case–control and cohort studies<br>Systematic reviews and meta-analyses<br>Phase III clinical trials | (Järvinen et al., 2000; de Jong et al., 2006)<br>(Bonis et al., 2007; Palomaki et al., 2009) |
| T3 | Guidelines to health practice | Surveys<br>Pilot studies<br>Phase IV clinical trials (also T4) | (Watkins et al., 2011)<br>(Hampel and de la Chapelle, 2011) |
| T4 | Practice to population health impact | Registries, surveys, surveillance<br>Economic analyses | (Campitelli et al., 2011)<br>(Mvundura et al., 2010) |

database added more than 8.2 million publications, of which 1.3 million (16%) are retrieved by searching for "gene" OR "genetic" OR "genome" OR "genomic" (NLM, 2012). Only about half of these articles involve humans, however, and many of these focus at the level of human genes, genomes, cells, or tissues, rather than human populations.

The basic science of public health genomics is human genome epidemiology, which offers an approach to population-level inference from genomic discoveries. This approach includes replicating and characterizing newly discovered genetic associations, describing the prevalence of genetic risk factors in different populations, assessing their contributions to disease burden, and evaluating gene–gene and gene–environment interactions (Khoury *et al.*, 2010b). The Human Genome Epidemiology Network (HuGENet; CDC, 2011) is a voluntary collaboration dedicated to developing reliable knowledge in this field by promoting standards for study conduct and reporting (Little *et al.*, 2009; Janssens *et al.*, 2011); developing tools for comprehensive literature searching (Yu *et al.*, 2008); improving synthesis of published and unpublished research data (Khoury *et al.*, 2009); and devising criteria for evaluating the evidence for genetic associations (Ioannidis *et al.*, 2008).

Bioinformatics has developed in parallel with molecular genetics as a science for organizing, archiving, visualizing, and sharing genomic data. The rapid growth of genotyping and sequencing capacity across the globe continues to stimulate the proliferation of genomic databases (see Chapter 9). Since 1996, the *Nucleic Acids Research* journal has published an annual database issue and compiled an online directory (Oxford Journals, 2012), which currently includes more than 1300 molecular biology databases (Galperin and Fernández-Suárez, 2012). The National Center for Biotechnology Information (NCBI, part of the National Library of Medicine) developed the Entrez search engine (NCBI, 2012) to connect a growing number of NCBI databases – extending from single nucleotide polymorphisms (SNPs) to genomes to genotypes from genome-wide association studies (GWAS) – within the vast knowledge context of PubMed.

The HuGE Navigator (HuGE Navigator, 2010) developed by Centers for Disease Control and Prevention (CDC)'s Office of Public Health Genomics, exploits NCBI infrastructure and common vocabularies such as HUGO and the Unified Medical Language System (UMLS) to create a comprehensive database of population-based epidemiologic studies of human genes (HUGO, 2012; NLM, 2009). The HuGE Navigator presents data extracted and curated from PubMed, along with a set of applications for searching and data mining (Yu *et al.*, 2008). The HuGE Navigator includes PubMed citations for more than 70,000 articles on genetic associations with a wide range of human diseases and traits. These include more than 1,200 published GWAS in the GWAS Catalog (National Human Genome Research Institute, 2012).

So far, most human genetic research in geographically or clinically defined human populations remains limited to such associations, which we classify as T1 on the translation continuum. For example, a 2007 analysis of publications in human genetics and genomics estimated that no more than 3% could be considered T2 or beyond (Khoury *et al.*, 2007). A comparable analysis in 2011, limited to cancer – one of the fastest-moving fields in genomic medicine – reached a similar conclusion (Schully *et al.*, 2012). For an example, see Box 11.1.

M. Gwinn and W.D. Dotson

## Box 11.1. Application: Genetic Associations with Lynch Syndrome

Lynch syndrome is an autosomal dominant condition that increases the risk of developing colorectal cancer, as well cancers at several other sites (e.g. endometrium, gastrointestinal tract, urinary tract). It is the most common cause of inherited colorectal cancer and accounts for approximately 3% of all colorectal cancer cases. It was first described in 1966 by Henry T. Lynch, who analyzed data from high-risk families (Lynch *et al.*, 1966) and coined the term hereditary non-polyposis colorectal cancer (HNPCC). Elucidating the underlying genetics entailed nearly 30 years of research on human germ line and tumor tissue and in model systems (OMIM, 2012). The observation of somatic changes in the length of repeat DNA sequences (microsatellite instability) led to the discovery of germline mutations in *MSH2* and *MLH1*, which are genes involved in DNA mismatch repair; together, they account for an estimated 90% of Lynch syndrome cases (OMIM, 2012). Mutations in at least ten other DNA mismatch repair genes have been implicated in smaller numbers of cases and additional genes have been studied as potential modifiers of the Lynch syndrome phenotype (e.g. cancer site and age of onset).

A search of the HuGE Navigator database for "Lynch syndrome" identifies more than 150 related publications since 2000, examining more than 70 different genes (Fig. 11.1). These articles include four meta-analyses and one GWAS (Giráldez *et al.*, 2012), which identified two novel loci associated with early-onset colorectal cancer.

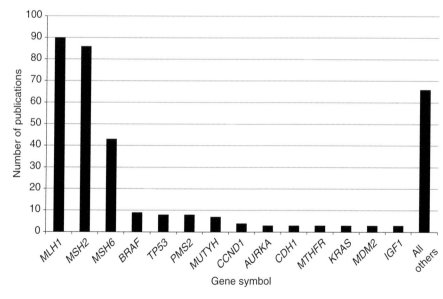

**Fig. 11.1.** Genes studied in relation to hereditary non-polyposis colorectal cancer (Lynch syndrome), HuGE Navigator (www.hugenavigator.net), July 2012.

## 11.3  T2: From Health Application to Evidence-based Guidelines

> [R]apid growth and potential does not mean that genomic tests
> should be issued a "pass" on the need for evidence.
> (Alfred O. Berg, 2009)

As part of the Human Genome Project, the National Institutes of Health (NIH)-Department of Energy (DOE) Working Group on Ethical, Legal, and Social Implications (ELSI) of Human Genome Research convened a Task Force on Genetic Testing to help guide the development of safe and effective genetic tests for use in clinical practice. In its final report, the Task Force defined three criteria for evaluating genetic tests: analytical validity, clinical validity, and clinical utility (Holtzman and Watson, 1997). To explain these concepts, it is helpful to consider a hypothetical test involving a single genetic variant. The "assay" is the laboratory method for determining the genotype; the "genetic test" is a process that includes the assay along with the information obtained from it (in this case, the genotype) and its interpretation (e.g. a risk level based on the measured genotype).

- Analytic validity is the accuracy and reliability of the assay in detecting the genotype, including its sensitivity and specificity in a set of well-defined samples.
- Clinical validity is the accuracy and consistency of the genetic test in predicting the associated phenotype, based on its clinical sensitivity, specificity, and predictive value.
- Clinical utility is a measure of the ability of the genetic test to lead to improved health outcomes, such as meaningful reductions in morbidity or mortality.

The ACCE (*Analytic validity, Clinical validity, Clinical Utility, and ELSI*) project, sponsored by CDC from 2000 to 2004, developed a systematic process for evaluating novel genetic tests based on these criteria (CDC, 2010). The ACCE model is flexible enough to apply to a broad range of emerging genomic applications, such as tests based on gene expression or epigenetic profiling.

Methods for the systematic review of evidence, including meta-analysis, are fundamental to developing guidelines for the use of proposed clinical interventions. The well-known Cochrane Collaboration maintains an extensive library of systematic reviews that are international in scope and conducted according to rigorous quality standards (Cochrane Collaboration, 2012). Although the Cochrane library includes genetic disorders as a topic area, its reviews focus on Mendelian disorders such as cystic fibrosis, sickle cell disease, and inborn errors of metabolism. Professional organizations such as the American College of Medical Genetics (ACMG) also produce clinical practice guidelines for diagnosis of rare, single-gene disorders (ACMG, 2012). CDC launched the Evaluation of Genomic Applications in Practice and Prevention (EGAPP) initiative in 2004 to develop and assess systematic methods for evaluating genetic tests relevant to more common, complex conditions (EGAPP, 2009; Teutsch *et al.*, 2009). Unlike most other evidence review processes, EGAPP considers observational (and, in some cases, unpublished) data because so few relevant data are available from randomized controlled trials. The EGAPP Working Group has further developed this approach and applied it to evaluate the evidence for several genetic tests; so far, only one evaluation has found sufficient evidence to make a positive recommendation, as described in Box 11.2 (EGAPP Working Group, 2009).

M. Gwinn and W.D. Dotson

Genetic tests may pose special challenges for evaluation because genetic assays and testing algorithms are often complex; furthermore, outcomes of their use may include implications not only for the person being tested but for family members (Botkin *et al.*, 2010). The US regulatory environment surrounding new genetic tests is

---

**Box 11.2. Application: Evidence for Cascade Screening of Relatives of Persons with Colorectal Cancer Related to Lynch Syndrome**

In 2009, the EGAPP Working Group recommended offering genetic testing for Lynch syndrome to all persons with newly diagnosed colorectal cancer as a strategy for reducing morbidity and mortality in their relatives (EGAPP Working Group, 2009). They reviewed a "chain of evidence" to conclude that offering relatives of these patients genetic testing – and where indicated, colorectal and endometrial cancer surveillance – could be expected to improve health outcomes. This approach, known as cascade screening, is illustrated in Fig. 11.2.

The evidence considered by the EGAPP Working Group was also published in two systematic reviews, which addressed questions related to analytic validity, clinical validity, and clinical utility (Bonis *et al.*, 2007; Palomaki *et al.*, 2009). These reviews identified many gaps in the published literature. For example, the EGAPP Working Group evaluated several different genetic tests – including preliminary tests (microsatellite instability, immunohistochemical staining, *BRAF* mutations) and diagnostic tests (genetic tests for DNA variants, including sequence changes and deletions) – but found insufficient evidence to recommend specific tests alone or in combination.

The evidence for clinical utility included seven studies describing uptake of counseling, testing, and colonoscopic surveillance among relatives. A non-randomized follow-up study of relatives of patients diagnosed with Lynch syndrome found a 62% reduction in colorectal cancer risk among those undergoing surveillance (Järvinen *et al.*, 2000). In addition, a cohort study among 146 families affected by Lynch syndrome found standardized mortality ratios of 6.5 for relatives undergoing colonoscopic surveillance, compared with 23.9 for those not undergoing surveillance (de Jong *et al.*, 2006).

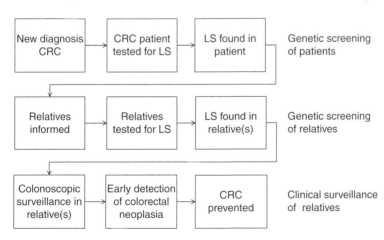

**Fig. 11.2.** Cascade screening to detect Lynch syndrome in relatives of persons with newly diagnosed colorectal cancer. CRC, colorectal cancer; LS, Lynch syndrome.

---

complicated, with laboratory developed tests (LDTs) and their components under the separate purviews of the Clinical Laboratory Improvement Acts of 1988 (CLIA) and the Food and Drug Administration (FDA), respectively. Regulatory reviews tend to focus on aspects of analytic and clinical validity, rather than on clinical utility. EGAPP was designed as a non-regulatory entity, similar to groups such as the US Preventive Services Task Force (USPSTF) and the Guide to Community Preventive Services (Community Guide), with an independent working group of non-federal employees developing optional guidelines or recommendations.

The EGAPP approach is designed to encompass testing applications across a broad range of medical specialties, focusing on tests that have potential public health impact. Several other groups – including consortia, such as the Clinical Pharmacogenetics Implementation Consortium (CPIC); professional organizations, such as the National Comprehensive Cancer Network (NCCN) and the American Society for Clinical Oncology (ASCO); and federally sponsored initiatives, such as the Secretary's Advisory Committee on Heritable Disorders in Newborns and Children (SACHDNC) – develop guidelines pertaining to genetic tests in their areas of specialization, often based on systematic reviews (Winn *et al.*, 1996; Calonge *et al.*, 2010; Relling and Klein, 2011; ASCO, 2012). A goal of those who hope to improve and expand the application of evidence-based methods in genetics has been to develop evidentiary standards that can be agreed upon by guideline developers from a broad range of application areas. Harmonization of methods would help promote the development of guidelines that are more consistent and easier to understand, and thus more useful to practitioners and the patient community (IOM, 2011).

## 11.4   T3: From Guidelines to Health Practice

> [I]f it is an evidence-based practice, where's the practice-based evidence?
>
> (Lawrence W. Green, 2008)

Although many genetic tests and other genomic applications have already entered the marketplace (and many more are on the way), very few evidence-based guidelines are available to support their use. An evolving, web-based table illustrates this "evidence gap" (Khoury *et al.*, 2011; CDC, 2012). Even when recommendations are available, however, there is no guarantee that their implementation in practice will be successful. A third phase of translation research (T3) examines factors affecting the successful dissemination and uptake of evidence-based recommendations into clinical practice and public health programs (see Box 11.3).

A recent Institute of Medicine report, *Clinical Practice Guidelines We Can Trust*, discussed standards for developing clinical practice guidelines and promoting their adoption (IOM, 2011). An important recommendation was to structure the format, vocabulary, and content of guidelines in ways that would allow them to be smoothly integrated into electronic clinical decision support. Additional factors affecting the uptake of evidence-based recommendations include social, economic, political, and other contextual issues. It has been suggested that implementation of research into practice depends equally upon "... the level and nature of the evidence, the context or environment into which the research is to be placed, and the method or way in which the process is facilitated" (Kitson *et al.*, 1998). Accordingly, T3 research reaches across multiple disciplines, including epidemiology.

M. Gwinn and W.D. Dotson

Qualitative research methods, such as focus groups and purposive sample surveys, can take on increased importance in T3 studies, for example, by engaging and surveying relevant stakeholders to identify end-users, along with their needs and preferences. Nevertheless, investigation of many important factors required for effective uptake, such as determinants of clinicians' awareness of a test, may be relatively easily addressed using quantitative epidemiologic surveys (Khoury et al., 2010a). Systematic reviews and meta-analyses of T3 "implementation science" are also gaining traction (Baskerville et al., 2012), allowing development of evidence-based intervention guidelines (Brouwers et al., 2011). A recent proposal for broadening and strengthening T3 research approaches emphasized five "core values": rigor and relevance, efficiency, collaboration, improved capacity, and cumulative knowledge (Glasgow et al., 2012).

---

**Box 11.3. Application: Implementing Universal Screening for Lynch Syndrome in Persons Newly Diagnosed with Colorectal Cancer**

Following publication of the EGAPP Working Group recommendation (EGAPP Working Group, 2009), the CDC convened a meeting in 2010 to explore approaches to implementing universal screening for Lynch syndrome in persons newly diagnosed with colorectal cancer (Bellcross et al., 2012). A preliminary analysis suggested that up to 5,000 colorectal cancers could be prevented in first- and second-degree relatives of these persons by cascade screening followed by colonoscopic surveillance at 1–3-year intervals of those at risk.

Meeting participants represented a variety of organizations, both public and private, and brought perspectives from a range of disciplines, including clinical genetics professionals, non-genetic clinicians, and epidemiologists. They discussed several existing, hospital-based programs that already offer universal screening for Lynch syndrome in persons diagnosed with colorectal cancer and highlighted a number of potential opportunities and challenges. Some of these are summarized in Table 11.2.

**Table 11.2.** Potential opportunities and challenges in implementing universal screening for Lynch syndrome in persons newly diagnosed with colorectal cancer (adapted from Bellcross et al., 2012).

| Opportunities | Challenges |
| --- | --- |
| More sensitive than screening based on family history criteria | Testing is complex and accuracy is not perfect |
| Testing and counseling can be centralized | Coordination among providers (e.g. pathologist, oncologist, genetic counselor) is required |
| Information technology can help with decision support and tracking | Non-genetic providers may lack knowledge of Lynch syndrome and testing issues |
| Relatives can benefit from testing, monitoring, and early intervention | Responsibility for informing relatives is not clear; effective strategies are needed |

---

## 11.5 T4: From Practice to Population Health Impact

Let's be realistic: If we didn't do it with aspirin, how can we expect to do it with DNA?
(Claude Lenfant, 2003)

Evidence-based guidelines are based on epidemiologic studies that demonstrate the efficacy of an intervention. Its effectiveness once in use in the "real" world, however, depends on many other factors, including characteristics of the population, clinical and public health practice, and social and environmental conditions. For example, the available evidence may be limited to observations of groups with more homogeneous clinical, demographic, or socioeconomic characteristics than the target population. Variations in practice also affect the population-level improvements in health outcomes that can be attributed to implementing evidence-based recommendations. Variations in the collection and coding of health data complicate reliable measurements, especially in a country such as the USA, in which most medical care is private and public health programs are delivered at the state level. In general, monitoring the population-level health benefits and risks (including morbidity and mortality) that result from a change in practice requires aligning the monitored population with that eligible for treatment. When these populations are only approximately similar, differences between them can lead to inaccurate or biased assessments.

Even in the highly variable US health care environment, some settings provide a basis for monitoring the health impact of genomic health applications. For example, health maintenance organizations (HMOs) can play a key role in evidence-based genomic medicine because they are able to institute standard practice guidelines and to monitor patient outcomes in a systematic way. In this setting, the relationship between evidence synthesis and evidence-based practice is bidirectional and dynamic because data on health outcomes (effectiveness) and the costs of implementation become part of the evidence base for decision making (IOM, 2009). Pharmacogenetic testing – the use of genetic information to predict response to drugs and guide therapy – is one of the most promising areas for study in HMOs and is an ongoing interest of the HMO Research Network (HMORN, 2012). The development of large, institutional biobanks linked to electronic medical records provides another potential setting for pharmacogenetic studies (Wilke and Dolan, 2011). For example, the NIH-sponsored Electronic Medical Records and Genomics (eMERGE) Network supports gene discovery research at clinical centers that maintain DNA biorepositories integrated with electronic medical records (eMERGE Network, 2012). In the future, such infrastructure could also serve in evaluating the use of genomic health applications that have entered clinical practice.

Genetically directed preventive interventions are more challenging to evaluate than those used to guide treatment. So far, the only genetic tests with sufficient predictive value for adult-onset diseases are for inherited forms of common, chronic conditions caused by genes with incomplete penetrance, such as those implicated in Lynch syndrome (see Box 11.4). Because these conditions are rare – accounting for only a small fraction of all cases of the disease in a population – it is difficult to accrue sufficient evidence for effectiveness. One approach to this problem is the use of registries, which have served a crucial role in developing and evaluating guidelines for managing childhood-onset genetic disorders, such as cystic fibrosis (Glauser *et al.*, 2012; Tangpricha *et al.*, 2012). Registries for familial, adult-onset diseases – such as the Breast and Colon Cancer Family Registries of the National Cancer Institute – have typically been established to support basic research; however, these registries can also support site-specific evaluations of guidelines and health impact (Campitelli *et al.*, 2011; NCI, 2012).

---

**Box 11.4. Application: Modeling Outcomes Associated with Lynch Syndrome Testing Strategies**

Cost-effectiveness analysis is an approach to knowledge synthesis focused on health outcomes, especially on comparing outcomes of alternative approaches to screening, diagnosis, or treatment. It differs from comparative effectiveness analysis by ascribing explicit economic values to both benefits and harms. A cost-effectiveness analysis compared the expected outcomes of four different testing algorithms for Lynch syndrome applied to a hypothetical population of patients with newly diagnosed colorectal cancer (Mvundura *et al.*, 2010). The main outcomes evaluated for each strategy were the total costs of testing, surveillance, and treatment for colorectal cancer in relatives and the expected numbers of life-years saved.

A sensitivity analysis was performed to assess the variability in expected outcomes that could be attributed to uncertainty in several key model inputs. The relative contribution of uncertainty associated with these inputs is summarized in Fig. 11.3, which is based on a scenario analysis described by Mvundura *et al.* (2010), which allowed inputs to vary in only one direction. Most inputs were varied in the direction of decreased cost; however, increased costs were modeled for four test-related inputs. In Fig. 11.3, all are represented by their absolute values. Note that inputs based on epidemiologic data tended to contribute much more uncertainty to the model than did inputs related to test performance.

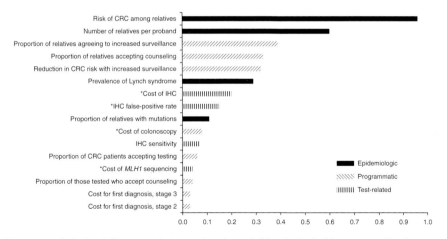

**Fig. 11.3.** Relative influence of uncertainty in variables included in a cost-effectiveness analysis of genetic testing strategies for Lynch syndrome (adapted from Mvundura *et al.*, 2010). Bar length represents relative absolute value; *indicates variables allowed to vary in a positive direction (others were allowed to vary in a negative direction only). CRC, colorectal cancer; IHC, immunohistochemistry.

---

## 11.6 Conclusion

> Translational epidemiology provides the key data needed to document what we
> know and what we do not know, and what works and what does not work,
> thus influencing further research, practice, and policy development.
>
> (Muin J. Khoury, 2010)

During the 20th century, genetics and epidemiology developed as largely separate sciences and their intersection, genetic epidemiology, remained a specialty focused on inherited diseases. Recently, however, genetics and epidemiology have undergone a form of convergent evolution, guided by advances in molecular biology, informatics, and statistics. The genes associated with more than 2,800 rare, inherited diseases are already mapped and nearly 2000 clinical tests for them are now available. Epidemiologic studies have also reliably documented several thousand genetic associations with common, complex diseases and traits; because the observed effects are mostly small, these discoveries do not translate directly into predictive or diagnostic tests.

Genetic epidemiology is currently well positioned to span biomedical and population-based health research by integrating genetic information with data on other biological, behavioral, environmental, and social characteristics. Translating this research presents a new opportunity to bridge clinical medicine with public health, by extending prevention and treatment beyond individuals to families and communities (Omenn, 2002). Translation is already well underway for some clinically recognized familial conditions such as Lynch syndrome, in which genetic testing can predict risk in affected families and guide preventive interventions. Indeed, studies of inherited forms of common diseases can offer insight into prevention strategies, even when specific genetic contributions to non-familial cases remain unknown. For example, although previous studies had suggested that aspirin protected against development of colorectal adenomas, the Colorectal Adenoma/carcinoma Prevention Program 2 (CAPP2) study of aspirin in Lynch syndrome was the first randomized clinical trial to demonstrate the protective effect of aspirin with colorectal cancer as an endpoint (Burn *et al.*, 2011). An accompanying editorial in *Lancet* observed that the results not only offered a strong argument for aspirin prophylaxis in Lynch syndrome, they "are also invaluable for the continued assessment of aspirin for prevention of sporadic colorectal cancer" (Chan and Lippman, 2011).

Epidemiologic methods are indispensable for evaluating the validity and utility of applications of genomic research proposed for use in healthcare. In most respects, these methods are the same as for other health-related applications and "genetic exceptionalism" is not warranted (Zimmern and Khoury, 2012). On the other hand, the appropriate use of genetic tests for risk assessment and counseling of relatives is difficult in a medical insurance system that is oriented to individuals rather than to extended families and communities. Perhaps our evolving understanding of the genetic architecture of the human population, which includes genetic variants rare and common, large and small, manifest and subtle, will help change our outlook on medicine and public health as well (Lupski *et al.*, 2011). Instead of setting "every man for himself" against "one size fits all," perhaps we can shape approaches to improving health that build on our networks of biological and social relationships.

M. Gwinn and W.D. Dotson

# Acknowledgment

The authors have no competing interests to declare.

# Further Reading

Green, E.D. and Guyer, M.S., National Human Genome Research Institute (2011) Charting a course for genomic medicine from base pairs to bedside. *Nature* 470, 204–213.

Khoury, M.J., Bedrosian, S.R., Gwinn, M., Higgins, J.P.T., Ioannidis, J.P.A. and Little, J. (eds) (2010) *Human Genome Epidemiology: Building the Evidence for Using Genetic Information to Improve Health and Prevent Disease,* 2nd edn. Oxford University Press, New York. Selected chapters available from: http://www.cdc.gov/genomics/resources/ books/2010_HuGE/index.htm (accessed July 19, 2012).

Khoury, M.J., Gwinn, M., Bowen, M.S. and Dotson, W.D. (2012) Beyond base pairs to bedside: a population perspective on how genomics can improve health. *American Journal of Public Health* 102, 34–37.

Teutsch, S.M., Bradley, L.A., Palomaki, G.E., Haddow, J.E., Piper, M., Calonge, N., *et al.* (2009) The Evaluation of Genomic Applications in Practice and Prevention (EGAPP) Initiative: methods of the EGAPP Working Group. *Genetics in Medicine* 11, 3–14.

# References

American College of Medical Genetics (ACMG) (2012) American College of Medical Genetics and Genomics Practice Guidelines. Available from: http://www.acmg.net/AM/Template. cfm?Section=Practice_Guidelines&Template=/CM/HTMLDisplay.cfm&ContentID=6821 (accessed July 20, 2012).

American Society of Clinical Oncology (ASCO) (2012) Practice & Guidelines. Available from: http://www.asco.org/ASCOv2/Practice+%26+Guidelines (accessed July 20, 2012).

Baskerville, N.B., Liddy, C. and Hogg, W. (2012) Systematic review and meta-analysis of practice facilitation within primary care settings. *Annals of Family Medicine* 10, 63–74.

Bellcross, C.A., Bedrosian, S.R., Daniels, E., Duquette, D., Hampel, H., Jasperson, K., *et al.* (2012) Implementing screening for Lynch syndrome among patients with newly diagnosed colorectal cancer: summary of a public health/clinical collaborative meeting. *Genetics in Medicine* 14, 152–162.

Berg, A.O. (2009) The CDC's EGAPP initiative: evaluating the clinical evidence for genetic tests. *American Family Physician* 80, 1218.

Bonis, P.A., Trikalinos, T.A., Chung, M., Chew, P., Ip, S., DeVine, D.A., *et al.* (2007) Hereditary nonpolyposis colorectal cancer: diagnostic strategies and their implications. *Evidence Report/Technology Assessment* 150, 1–180. Available from: http://www.ncbi.nlm.nih. gov/books/NBK38285/ (accessed July 19, 2012).

Botkin, J.R., Teutsch, S.M., Kaye, C.I., Hayes, M., Haddow, J.E., Bradley, L.A., *et al.* (2010) Outcomes of interest in evidence-based evaluations of genetic tests. *Genetics in Medicine* 12, 228–235.

Brouwers, M.C., De Vito, C., Bahirathan, L., Carol, A., Carroll, J.C. and Cotterchio, M. (2011) Effective interventions to facilitate the uptake of breast, cervical and colorectal cancer screening: an implementation guideline. *Implementation Science* 6, 112.

Burke, W., Khoury, M.J., Stewart, A. and Zimmern, R.L. (2006) The path from genome-based research to population health: development of an international public health genomics network. *Genetics in Medicine* 8, 451–458.

Burn, J., Gerdes, M.-A., Macrae, F., Mecklin, J.-P., Moeslein, G., Olschwang, S., *et al.* (2011) Long-term effect of aspirin on cancer risk in carriers of hereditary colorectal cancer: an analysis from the CAPP2 randomised controlled trial. *Lancet* 378, 2081–2087.

Calonge, N., Green, N.S., Rinaldo, P., Lloyd-Puryear, M., Dougherty, D., Boyle, C., *et al.* (2010) Committee report: method for evaluating conditions nominated for population-based screening of newborns and children. *Genetics in Medicine* 12, 153–159.

Campitelli, M., Chiarelli, A.M., Mirea, L., Stewart, L., Glendon, G., Ritvo, P., *et al.* (2011) Adherence to breast and ovarian cancer screening recommendations for female relatives from the Ontario site of the Breast Cancer Family Registry. *European Journal of Cancer Prevention* 20, 492–500.

Centers for Disease Control and Prevention (CDC) Public Health Genomics (2010) ACCE model process for evaluating genetic tests. Available from: http://www.cdc.gov/genomics/gtesting/ACCE/ (accessed July 20, 2012).

Centers for Disease Control and Prevention (CDC) Public Health Genomics (2011) Human Genome Epidemiology Network (HuGENet). Available from: http://www.cdc.gov/genomics/hugenet/ (accessed July 20, 2012).

Centers for Disease Control and Prevention (CDC) Public Health Genomics (2012) Genomic tests by levels of evidence. Available from: http://www.cdc.gov/genomics/gtesting/tier.htm (accessed July 20,2012).

Chan, A.T. and Lippman, S.M. (2011) Aspirin and colorectal cancer prevention in Lynch syndrome. *Lancet* 378, 2051–2052.

Cochrane Collaboration (2012) Cochrane reviews. Available from: http://www.cochrane.org/cochrane-reviews (accessed July 20, 2012).

Contopoulos-Ioannidis, D.G., Alexiou, G.A., Gouvias, T.C. and Ioannidis, J.P.A. (2008) Life cycle of translational research. *Science* 321, 1298–1299.

Cordell, H.J. and Clayton, D.G. (2005) Genetic association studies. *Lancet* 366, 1121–1131.

de Jong, A.E., Hendriks, Y.M., Kleibeuker, J.H., de Boerk, S.Y., Cats, A., Griffioen, G., *et al.* (2006) Decrease in mortality in Lynch syndrome families because of surveillance. *Gastroenterology* 130, 665–671.

eMERGE Network. (2012) Electronic medical records & genomics. Available from: https://www.mc.vanderbilt.edu/victr/dcc/projects/acc/index.php/Main_Page (accessed July 20, 2012).

Evaluation of Genomic Applications in Practice and Prevention (EGAPP) (2009) EGAPP reviews.org homepage. Available from: http://egappreviews.org/ (accessed July 20, 2012).

Evaluation of Genomic Applications in Practice and Prevention (EGAPP) Working Group (2009) Recommendations from the EGAPP Working Group: genetic testing strategies in newly diagnosed individuals with colorectal cancer aimed at reducing morbidity and mortality from Lynch syndrome in relatives. *Genetics in Medicine* 11, 35–41.

Galperin, M.Y. and Fernández-Suárez, X.M. (2012) The 2012 Nucleic Acids Research Database Issue and the online Molecular Biology Database Collection. *Nucleic Acids Research* 40, D1–D8.

Giráldez, M.D., López-Dóriga, A., Bujanda, L., Abulí, A., Bessa, X., Fernández-Rozadilla, C., *et al.* (2012) Susceptibility genetic variants associated with early-onset colorectal cancer. *Carcinogenesis* 33, 613–619.

Glasgow, R.E., Vinson, C., Chambers, D., Khoury, M.J., Kaplan, R.M. and Hunter, C. (2012) National Institutes of Health approaches to dissemination and implementation science: current and future directions. *American Journal of Public Health* 102, 1274–1281.

Glauser, T.A., Nevins, P.H., Williamson, J.C., Abdolrasulnia, M., Salinas, G.D., Zhang, J., *et al.* (2012) Adherence to the 2007 cystic fibrosis pulmonary guidelines: a national survey of CF care centers. *Pediatric Pulmonology* 47, 434–440.

Green, L.W. (2008) Making research relevant: if it is an evidence-based practice, where's the practice-based evidence? *Family Practice* 25, i20–24.

M. Gwinn and W.D. Dotson

Hampel, H. and de la Chapelle, A. (2011) The search for unaffected individuals with Lynch syndrome: do the ends justify the means? *Cancer Prevention Research* 4, 1–5.

HMO Research Network (HMORN) (2012) Welcome to the HMO Research Network. Available from: http://www.hmoresearchnetwork.org/ (accessed July 20, 2012).

Holtzman, N.A. and Watson, M.S. (eds) (1997) Promoting Safe and Effective Testing in the United States. Final Report of the Task Force on Genetic Testing. National Human Genome Research Institute, Bethesda, Maryland. Available from: http://www.genome.gov/10001733 (accessed July 19, 2012).

HuGE Navigator (2010) HuGE Navigator version 2.0, an integrated, searchable knowledge base of genetic associations and human genome epidemiology. Available from: http://www.hugenavigator.net/HuGENavigator/home.do (accessed 20 July 2012).

HUGO (2012) HUGO Gene Nomenclature Committee (HGNC) genenames.org homepage. Available from: http://www.genenames.org/ (accessed July 20, 2012).

Institute of Medicine (IOM) National Research Council (2009) *Systems for Research and Evaluation for Translating Genome-Based Discoveries for Health: Workshop Summary.* The National Academies Press, Washington, DC.

Institute of Medicine (IOM) National Research Council (2011) *Clinical Practice Guidelines We Can Trust.* The National Academies Press, Washington, DC.

Ioannidis, J.P.A., Boffetta, P., Little, J., O'Brien, T.R., Uitterlinden, A.G., Vineis, P., *et al.* (2008) Assessment of cumulative evidence on genetic associations: interim guidelines. *International Journal of Epidemiology* 37, 120–132.

Järvinen, H.J., Aarnio, M., Mustonen, H., Aktan-Collan, K., Aaltonen, L.A., Peltomäki, P., *et al.* (2000) Controlled 15-year trial on screening for colorectal cancer in families with hereditary nonpolyposis colorectal cancer. *Gastroenterology* 118, 829–834.

Janssens, A.C.W., Ioannidis, J.P.A., van Duijn, C.M., Little, J. Khoury, M.J., *et al.* (2011) Strengthening the reporting of genetic risk prediction studies: the GRIPS Statement. *PLoS Medicine* 8, e1000420.

Khoury, M.J., Gwinn, M., Yoon, P.W., Dowling, N., Moore, C.A. and Bradley L. (2007) The continuum of translation research in genomic medicine: how can we accelerate the appropriate integration of human genome discoveries into health care and disease prevention? *Genetics in Medicine* 9, 665–674.

Khoury, M.J., Bertram, L., Boffetta, P., Butterworth, A.S., Chanock, S.J., Dolan, S.M., *et al.* (2009) Genome-wide association studies, field synopses, and the development of the knowledge base on genetic variation and human diseases. *American Journal of Epidemiology* 170, 269–279.

Khoury, M.J., Gwinn, M. and Ioannidis, J.P.A. (2010a) The emergence of translational epidemiology: from scientific discovery to population health impact. *American Journal of Epidemiology* 172, 517–524.

Khoury, M.J., Bedrosian, S.R., Gwinn, M., Higgins, J.P.T., Ioannidis, J.P.A. and Little, J. (eds) (2010b) *Human Genome Epidemiology: Building the Evidence for Using Genetic Information to Improve Health and Prevent Disease*, 2nd edn. Oxford University Press, New York. Selected chapters available from: http://www.cdc.gov/genomics/resources/books/2010_HuGE/index.htm (accessed July 19, 2012).

Khoury, M.J., Bowen, M.S., Burke, W., Coates, R.J., Dowling, N.F., Evans, J. P., *et al.* (2011) Current priorities for public health practice in addressing the role of human genomics in improving population health. *American Journal of Preventive Medicine* 40, 486–493.

Kitson, A., Harvey, G. and McCormack, B. (1998) Enabling the implementation of evidence based practice: a conceptual framework. *Quality Health Care* 7, 149–158.

Lenfant, C. (2003) Clinical research to clinical practice – lost in translation? *New England Journal of Medicine* 349, 868–874.

Little, J., Higgins, J.P.T., Ioannidis, J.P.A., Moher, D., Gagnon, F., von Elm, E., *et al.* (2009) STrengthening the REporting of Genetic Association Studies (STREGA): an extension of the STROBE statement. *PLoS Medicine* 6, e22.

Lupski, J.R., Belmont, J.W., Boerwinkle, E. and Gibbs, R.A. (2011) Clan genomics and the complex architecture of human disease. *Cell* 147, 32–43.

Lynch, H.T., Shaw, M.W., Magnuson, C.W., Larsen, A.L. and Krush, A.J. (1966) Hereditary factors in cancer. Study of two large Midwestern kindreds. *Archives of Internal Medicine* 117, 206–212.

Mvundura, M., Grosse, S.D., Hampel, H. and Palomaki, G.E. (2010) The cost-effectiveness of genetic testing strategies for Lynch syndrome among newly diagnosed patients with colorectal cancer. *Genetics in Medicine* 12, 93–104.

National Cancer Institute (NCI) (2012) Breast and colon cancer family registries. Available from: http://epi.grants.cancer.gov/CFR/ (accessed July 20, 2012).

National Center for Biotechnology Information (NCBI) (2012) Entrez, the life sciences search engine. Available from: http://www.ncbi.nlm.nih.gov/sites/gquery (accessed July 20, 2012).

National Human Genome Research Institute (2012) Hindorff, L.A., MacArthur, J., Wise, A., Junkins, H.A., Hall, P.N., Klemm, A.K. and Manolio, T.A. A catalog of published genome-wide association studies. Available from: www.genome.gov/gwastudies (accessed July 19, 2012).

National Library of Medicine (NLM) (2009) Unified Medical Language System® [UMLS®]. Available from: http://www.nlm.nih.gov/research/umls/ (accessed July 20, 2012).

National Library of Medicine (NLM) (2012) PubMed. Available from: www.ncbi.nlm.nih.gov/pubmed/ (accessed July 20, 2012).

Omenn, G.S. (2002) The crucial role of the public health sciences in the postgenomic era. *Genetics in Medicine* 4, 21S–26S.

Online Mendelian Inheritance in Man (OMIM) (2012) Lynch syndrome I (#120435). Available from: http://www.omim.org/entry/120435 (accessed July 19, 2012).

Oxford Journals (2012) *Nucleic Acids Research*, 2012 NAR database summary paper alphabetic list. Available from: http://www.oxfordjournals.org/nar/database/a/ (accessed July 20, 2012).

Palomaki, G.E., McClain, M.R., Melillo, S., Hampel, H.L. and Thibodeau, S.N. (2009) EGAPP supplementary evidence review: DNA testing strategies aimed at reducing morbidity and mortality from Lynch syndrome. *Genetics in Medicine* 11, 42–65.

Relling, M.V. and Klein, T.E. (2011) CPIC: Clinical Pharmacogenetics Implementation Consortium of the Pharmacogenomics Research Network. *Clinical Pharmacology and Therapeutics* 89, 464–467.

Schully, S.D., Benedicto, C.B. and Khoury, M.J. (2012) How can we stimulate translational research in cancer genomics beyond bench to bedside? *Genetics in Medicine* 14, 169–170.

Tangpricha, V., Kelly, A, Stephenson, A., Maguiness, K., Enders, J., Robinson, K.A., *et al.* (2012) An update on the screening, diagnosis, management, and treatment of vitamin D deficiency in individuals with cystic fibrosis: evidence-based recommendations from the Cystic Fibrosis Foundation. *Journal of Clinical Endocrinology and Metabolism* 97, 1082–1093.

Teutsch, S.M., Bradley, L.A., Palomaki, G.E., Haddow, J.E., Piper, M., Calonge, N., *et al.* (2009) The Evaluation of Genomic Applications in Practice and Prevention (EGAPP) Initiative: methods of the EGAPP Working Group. *Genetics in Medicine* 11, 3–14.

Thomas, D.C. (2000) Genetic epidemiology with a capital "E". *Genetic Epidemiology* 19, 289–300.

Watkins, K.E., Way, C.Y., Fiander, J.J., Meadus, R.J., Esplen, M.J., Green, J.S., *et al.* (2011) Lynch syndrome: barriers to and facilitators of screening and disease management. *Hereditary Cancer in Clinical Practice* 9, 8.

Watson, P. and Lynch, H.T. (2001) Cancer risk in mismatch repair gene mutation carriers. *Familial Cancer* 1, 57–60.

White, K.L. (1991) *Healing the Schism: Epidemiology, Medicine, and the Public's Health.* Springer-Verlag, New York.

Wilke, R.A. and Dolan, M.E. (2011) Genetics and variable drug response. *JAMA* 306, 306–307.

Winn, R.J., Botnick, W. and Dozier, N. (1996) The NCCN Guidelines Development Program. *Oncology (Williston Park).* 10 (11 Suppl.), 23–28.

Yu, W., Gwinn, M., Clyne, M., Yesupriya, A. and Khoury, M.J. (2008) A navigator for human genome epidemiology. *Nature Genetics* 40, 124–125.

Zimmern, R.L. and Khoury, M.J. (2012) The impact of genomics on public health practice: the case for change. *Public Health Genomics* 15, 118–124.

# Index

Note: page numbers in *italics* refer to figures and tables, those in **bold** refer to boxes